CLINICAL AND EXPERIMENTAL PATHOLOGY OF LUNG CANCER

DEVELOPMENTS IN ONCOLOGY

F.J. Cleton and J.W.I.M. Simons, eds., Genetic Origins of Tumour Cells. ISBN 90-247-2272-1
J. Aisner and P. Chang, eds., Cancer Treatment Research. ISBN 90-247-2358-2
B.W. Ongerboer de Visser, D.A. Bosch and W.M.H. van Woerkom-Eykenboom, eds., Neuro-oncology: Clinical and Experimental Aspects. ISBN 90-247-2421-X
K. Hellmann, P. Hilgard and S. Eccles, eds., Metastasis: Clinical and Experimental Aspects. ISBN 90-247-2424-4
H.F. Seigler, ed., Clinical Management of Melanoma. ISBN 90-247-2584-4
P. Correa and W. Haenszel, eds., Epidemiology of Cancer of the Digestive Tract. ISBN 90-247-2601-8
L.A. Liotta and I.R. Hart, eds., Tumour Invasion and Metastasis. ISBN 90-247-2611-5
J. Bánóczy, ed., Oral Leukoplakia. ISBN 90-247-2655-7
C. Tijssen, M. Halprin and L. Endtz, eds., Familial Brain Tumours. ISBN 90-247-2691-3
F.M. Muggia, C.W. Young and S.K. Carter, eds., Anthracycline Antibiotics in Cancer. ISBN 90-247-2711-1
B.W. Hancock, ed., Assessment of Tumour Response. ISBN 90-247-2712-X
D.E. Peterson, ed., Oral Complications of Cancer Chemotherapy. ISBN 0-89838-563-6
R. Mastrangelo, D.G. Poplack and R. Riccardi, eds., Central Nervous System Leukemia. Prevention and Treatment. ISBN 0-89838-570-9
A. Polliack, ed., Human Leukemias. Cytochemical and Ultrastructural Techniques in Diagnosis and Research. ISBN 0-89838-585-7
W. Davis, C. Maltoni and S. Tanneberger, eds., The Control of Tumor Growth and its Biological Bases. ISBN 0-89838-603-9
A.P.M. Heintz, C.Th. Griffiths and J.B. Trimbos, eds., Surgery in Gynecological Oncology. ISBN 0-89838-604-7
M.P. Hacker, E.B. Double and I. Krakoff, eds., Platinum Coordination Complexes in Cancer Chemotherapy. ISBN 0-89838-619-5
M.J. van Zwieten, The Rat as Animal Model in Breast Cancer Research: A Histopathological Study of Radiation- and Hormone-Induced Rat Mammary Tumors. ISBN 0-89838-624-1
B. Löwenberg and A. Hagenbeek, eds., Minimal Residual Disease in Acute Leukemia. ISBN 0-89838-630-6
I. van der Waal and G.B. Snow, eds., Oral Oncology. ISBN 0-89838-631-4
B.W. Hancock and A.H. Ward, eds., Immunological Aspects of Cancer. ISBN 0-89838-664-0
K.V. Honn and B.F. Sloane, Hemostatic Mechanisms and Metastasis. ISBN 0-89838-667-5
K.R. Harrap, W. Davis and A.H. Calvert, eds., Cancer Chemotherapy and Selective Drug Development. ISBN 0-89838-673-3
C.J.H. van de Velde and P.H. Sugarbaker, eds., Liver Metastasis. ISBN 0-89838-648-5
D.J. Ruiter, K. Welvaart and S. Ferrone, eds., Cutaneous Melanoma and Precursor Lesions. ISBN 0-89838-689-6
S.B. Howell, ed., Intra-arterial and Intracavitary Cancer Chemotherapy. ISBN 0-89838-691-8
D.L. Kisner and J.F. Smyth, eds., Interferon Alpha-2: Pre-Clinical and Clinical Evaluation. ISBN 0-89838-701-9
P. Furmanski, J.C. Hager and M.A. Rich, eds., RNA Tumor Viruses, Oncogenes, Human Cancer and Aids: On the Frontiers of Understanding. ISBN 0-89838-703-5
J. Talmadge, I.J. Fidler and R.K. Oldham, Screening for Biological Response Modifiers: Methods and Rationale. ISBN 0-89838-712-4
J.C. Bottino, R.W. Opfell and F.M. Muggia, eds., Liver Cancer. ISBN 0-89838-713-2
P.K. Pattengale, R.J. Lukes and C.R. Taylor, Lymphoproliferative Diseases: Pathogenesis, Diagnosis, Therapy. ISBN 0-89838-725-6
F. Cavalli, G. Bonadonna and M. Rozencweig, eds., Malignant Lymphomas and Hodgkin's Disease: Experimental and Therapeutic Advances. ISBN 0-89838-727-2
J.G. McVie, W. Bakker, Sj.Sc. Wagenaar and D. Carney, eds., Clinical and Experimental Pathology of Lung Cancer. ISBN 0-89838-764-7

CLINICAL AND EXPERIMENTAL PATHOLOGY OF LUNG CANCER

edited by

J.G. McVie
Netherlands Cancer Institute, Amsterdam, The Netherlands

W. Bakker
Department of Pneumology, University Hospital Leiden, The Netherlands

Sj.Sc. Wagenaar
Department of Pathological Anatomy, Sint Antonius Hospital, Nieuwegein, The Netherlands

D. Carney
Mater Miserecordia Hospital, Dublin, Ireland

1986 **MARTINUS NIJHOFF PUBLISHERS**
a member of the KLUWER ACADEMIC PUBLISHERS GROUP
DORDRECHT / BOSTON / LANCASTER

Distributors

for the United States and Canada: Kluwer Academic Publishers, 190 Old Derby Street, Hingham, MA 02043, USA
for the UK and Ireland: Kluwer Academic Publishers, MTP Press Limited, Falcon House, Queen Square, Lancaster LA1 1RN, UK
for all other countries: Kluwer Academic Publishers Group, Distribution Center, P.O. Box 322, 3300 AH Dordrecht, The Netherlands

Library of Congress Cataloging in Publication Data

```
Main entry under title:

Clinical and experimental pathology of lung cancer.

    (Developments in oncology)
    "Based upon a Boerhaave course organized by the
Faculty of Medicine, University of Leiden, The
Netherlands, in co-operation with the International
Association for the Study of Lung Cancer, and the
European Organization for Research on Treatment of
Cancer (EORTC)/Lung Cancer Cooperative Group"--
T.p. verso.
    Includes bibliographies and index.
    1. Lungs--Cancer--Congresses.  I. McVie, J. G.
II. Rijksuniversiteit te Leiden.  Faculteit der
Geneeskunde.   III. International Association for the
Study of Lung Cancer.  IV. European Organization for
Research on Treatment of Cancer.  Lung Cancer
Cooperative Group.  V. Series.  [DNLM: 1. Lung
Neoplasms--pathology--congresses.
W1 DE998N / WF 658 C641]
RC280.L8C55  1985       616.99'42407        85-21555
ISBN 0-89838-764-7 (U.S.)
```

ISBN 0-89838-764-7 (this volume)

Book information

This publication is based upon a Boerhaave course organized by the Faculty of Medicine, University of Leiden, The Netherlands, in co-operation with the International Association for the Study of Lung Cancer and the European Organization for Research on Treatment of Cancer (EORTC)/Lung Cancer Cooperative Group.

Copyright

PRINTED IN THE NETHERLANDS

PREFACE

J.G.MCVIE

The impact of therapy on one subset of lung cancer, the "small cell" type
has been significant and lasting. The reality of cure for even a fraction
of patients with this disease has caused reverberations in the pathology
lab where the responsibility and challenge of diagnosis of this vital sub
group lies. No less dramatic has been the discovery that the cell types of
lung cancer have recognisable growth characteristics in serum free culture,
they are recognisable by patterns of markers and some produce growth
factors which autoregulate their eventual fate. Many of the discoveries
from the biological studies have impacted on the pathologist in the form
of disturbing evidence for a single stem cell origin for all the cell types
of lung cancer and in the shape of new facilitation in diagnosis by application of immunoperoxidase techniques. Monoclonal antibodies raised against
oncogene products, growth factor receptor sites, "bystander" cell membrane
proteins can all be applied to cytology specimens and frozen or paraffin
fixed tissue sections to aid diagnosis and some can be used in sequential
serum assay to monitor therapy and predict prognosis.
Adding to these extraordinary tools, the sophistication of electron microscopy and immuno-electron microscopy, new techniques for preparation of
tissue and novel methods for studying vital cells in "kinesis", you sense
the flavour of the future of lung cancer which is captured in this book.
The accent in presenting the different facets of lung cancer research has
been firmly laid on the interface between basic scientist (chromosome man,
biologist, molecular biologist), the pathologist (skilled nowadays in
electron microscopy and immunodiagnostics) and the consumer (lung cancer
specialist be he surgeon, physician or radiotherapist). It is inconceivable
that this explosion of new ideas, backed by the required technology chanel-
led as it is now has been towards the patient, will not lead to attainment
of yet more distant goals - the increase in cure rate in small cell cancer
and the breakdown of the resistant barriers of non small cell types.

CONTENTS

VIII

LIST OF MAJOR CONTRIBUTORS

J.Aisner   Baltimore Cancer Research Center,
                            Baltimore, U.S.A.

W.Bakker   Dept.of Pneumology, University Hospital,
                            Leiden, The Netherlands

F.T.Bosman   Dept.of Pathology, State University,
                            Maastricht, The Netherlands

D.Carney   Mater Miserecordia Hospital, Dublin,
                            Ireland

B.Corrin   Dept.of Pathology, Brompton Hospital,
                            London, United Kingdom

A.J.van der Eb   Dept. of Medical Biochemistry, Sylvius
                            Laboratories, Leiden, The Netherlands

J.D.Elema   Dept.of Pathology, State University,
                            Groningen, The Netherlands

C.Gropp   Klinikum der Philipps Universität Marburg,
                            Marburg, West Germany

H.H.Hansen   Dept.of Chemotherapy, Finsen Institute,
                            Copenhagen, Denmark

F.R.Hirsch   Dept.of Chemotherapy R II, Finsen Institute,
                            Copenhagen, Denmark

W.W.Johnston   Duke University Medical Center,
                            Durham, U.S.A.

M.J.Matthews   NCI-Navy Medical Oncology Branch,
                            Bethesda, U.S.A.

J.G.McVie   Netherlands Cancer Institute,
                            Amsterdam, The Netherlands

R.K.Oldham   Biological Therapy Institute,
                            Franklin, Tennessee, U.S.A.

H.T.Planteydt   Dept.of Path.Anatomy, Bethesda-St.Joseph
                            Hospital, Vlissingen, The Netherlands

E.Roos   Netherlands Cancer Institute,
                            Amsterdam, The Netherlands

D.J.Ruiter   Dept.of Pathology, State University,
                            Leiden, The Netherlands

X

Y.Shimosato   Pathology Division, National Cancer Center
Research Institute, Tokyo, Japan

L.L.Vindeløv   Medical Dept., Finsen Institute,
Copenhagen, Denmark

Sj.Sc.Wagenaar   Dept.of Path.Anatomy, St.Antonius Hospital,
Nieuwegein, The Netherlands

L.B.Woolner   Dept.of Surgical Pathology, Mayo Clinics,
Rochester, U.S.A.

HISTOPATHOLOGIC TYPING OF LUNG CANCER.
Etiologic and epidemiologic features.

HEINE H. HANSEN

1.INTRODUCTION

Lung cancer has within the last decade emerged as one of the
biggest challenges in oncology. This challenge is caused both
by the continuing increasing rise in incidence in most developed countries and because there is an increase in the heavy
marketing of manufactured cigarettes in developing countries
thereby producing a large increase in lung cancer in those
countries in the early part of the next century. The increase
in the developed countries is particularly seen among younger
females, andthe increase is so large that in some countries,
including the U.S.A., as many females will die annually from
lung cancer as from breast cancer by 1990.
Within the last years the importance of a precise histologic
classification of lung cancer has been well established both
when etiologic, epidemiologic, biologic, diagnostic and therapeutic features of lung cancer are discussed. It is outside
the scope of this article to give an extensive review of all
these topics, some of which are presented elsewhere in this
book. Instead specific points will be discussed including the
relation between cell type and smoking, and the question
whether there has been a change in incidence of the various
cell types within the last decade.

2. CELL TYPE AND SMOKING

It is a common belief that here are more smokers in the squamous and small cell type (Kreyberg group 1) than in the adenocarcinoma cell type (Kreyberg group 2) as first pointed out
in the early 1960's. Since then reports by Wynder et
al. (1) and Yesner et al. (2) have supported this close association between squamous and small cell types and cigarette
smoking. Of interest is that Yesner et al. (2) in Kreyberg
type 1 found that the ratio of squamous cell type to small
cell carcinoma changed from 3-1 in light smokers to 3-2 in
moderate smokers to 3-3 in heavy smokers. The small cell carcinoma was thus the only histologic type which increased
linearly   with the amount smoked. Noteworthy is also the
observation that there was a slight increase in adenocarcinoma
from 19 to 27% from light to heavy smoking. Other data from the
region of Bern (3) and from a study by McD. Herrold (4) are
less convincing when relating certain cell types to the
amount of cigarette smoking. The latter analyzed histologic
material in 1477 of 2241 men registered as dying from lung

cancer among a total number of 46,270 deaths among U.S. veterans in the period 1954-1962. The investigator was unable to
confirm the sharp correlation between the amount of tobacco
smoked and the histologic cell types; even a significantly
greater proportion of group 1 tumors was observed in smokers
of cigarettes than among the non-smokers. The data from
Switzerland included 223 patients from the period 1974-1976
(figure 1). All patients were classified according to the 4
major histologic cell types using the WHO classification.
The study demonstrated that WHO types II, III and IV were seen
more often among persons from urban regions than squamous
cell carcinoma patients who were evenly distributed among the
rural and urban parts of the region of Bern.
The discrepancy between the various studies might be explained
by various factors such as
a) differences in the various histopathologic classifications
   applied,
b) differences in intra- and interobserver variability,
c) differences in material obtained for histopathologic
   typing (bronchial biopsy versus surgical biopsy versus
   autopsy material),
d) changes in the relative composition of the various
   carcinogens and co-carcinogens during the time period
   analyzed.

3.CHANGES IN THE INCIDENCE OF THE VARIOUS MAJOR HISTOLOGIC TYPES

Information from the literature concerning a possible change
in the incidence during a fixed time period is scarce and
again hampered by many of the factors outlined above. In addition the information obtained from various cancer registers
rarely includes the detailed information on the histopathologic
classification applied. Even when the latter information is
given a number of factors might influence the completeness
and reliability of such registrations, as illustrated
by Larsson (5). In a review of a cancer registry covering a
6-year period 988 cases of lung cancer in a geographic area
of 16,666 km^2 covering a population of 1,086,692 in the south-
west region of Sweden was reanalyzed including histopathologic
reclassification according to classification proposed by WHO
Reference Center in 1967. According to the registry the diagnosis had been based on positive histology in 94.7% and on
cytology in 2.5%. In the final revised series positive histology had been obtained in 96.8% and cytology in only 1.1%.
The frequency of microscopical confirmation was thus very high
and the completeness in reporting cases seems also to have
been very satisfactory. In contrast the registration of histologic types of primary lung cancer did not produce the desired
results. The recorded histologic diagnosis epidermoid carcinoma was correct in 77% of the cases, adenocarcinoma in 79% and
anaplastic in only 46% as per reclassification performed by
one experienced pathologist (table 1).

With respect to differences in the percentage of histopathologic distribution between various geographic areas it continues
to be difficult to obtain data truly representative not only
because of differences in histopathologic interpretation but
also because of the selection factor influencing the referral
of certain patient-groups with inclusion of certain cell
types but not others to major cancer centers. In table 2 the
distribution from various regions of the world is given.
In all studies the WHO classification of 1967 is applied but
even then the percentage distribution varies considerably.
It is evident, however, that epidermoid carcinoma is the most
frequently registered cell type with exception of Iceland where
small cell carcinoma is the dominating cell type.
Of special interest are the studies from Hong Kong performed
in the period 1960-1972 and 1973-1982 where an increase is
noted in the frequency of adenocarcinoma with a concomitant
decrease in the other cell types - a trend which has also been
observed by e.g. Vincent et al. analyzing 682 cases of lung
cancer registered between 1962-1975 at the Lung Cancer Tumor
Registry at the thoracic surgical department at Roswell Park
Memorial Institute, Buffalo, New York (10). Detailed analysis
of the data from Hong Kong reveals some interesting
points. In table 3 the data from the period 1960-1972 and
1973-1982 are given with distribution according to sex and
histologic types using the WHO 1967 classification. A direct
comparison is of interest because in addition to the same
classification both groups were based on autopsy data
coming from the same department with the same catchment area
having the same exclusion criteria. In addition the cohorts
had relatively large numbers of patients consisting of 853
and 1,055 cases respectively. From table 3 it is obvious
that there is an increase in proportion of adenocarcinoma in
the male from 15.6% to 25.8% (P < 0.02) and in the female
from 34.3% to 49.6% (p < 0.01).
The increase in adenocarcinoma is accompanied by a decrease
in percentage of squamous cell carcinoma but not of small cell
carcinoma in males. The opposite is true for the females.
The increase in adenocarcinoma is associated with decrease in
the small cell carcinoma but not in squamous cell carcinoma.
The proportion of large cell carcinoma remains constant in
both series. It is unlikely that there should be a significant
interobserver variation as the same classification is used.
The slides were reviewed blindly and the change noted was
seen in squamous cell, small cell and adenocarcinoma which
are unlikely to be confused with one another in contrast to
large cell carcinoma.
The same authors used the same material to make another interesting and important observation when they compared the
WHO 1967 and the WHO 1981 classification (table 4). The data
clearly indicate that the change of the WHO classification
per se results in a marked increase for adenocarcinoma with a
similar decrease for large cell carcinoma. The findings are as
expected according to the change in the definition of the 2
respective cell types in the 2 classifications.

4

In spite of the latter observation it is thus clear that there
is a definite tendency for adenocarcinoma to increase in
Hong Kong - a trend which as mentioned previously has also
been noted in the U.S.A. The studies from the U.S.A. further
suggest that the increase is mainly due to an increase in
females while the studies from Hong Kong report increase in
both sexes.
This change in histopathologic pattern of lung cancer is
important and raises many questions such as whether the same
etiologic agents operate in both men and females or whether
there are also genetic factors influencing the development
of the various cell types.
It is obvious that carefully planned epidemiologic prospective studies with detailed analysis are needed,based on
universally acceptable uniform methods for histological classification of lung cancer with material of similar source
and detailed information concerning intra- and interobserver
variability. Hopefully, such data will be obtained within the
next decade, thereby adding additional information to the
epidemiology of the various types of lung cancer.

REFERENCES

1. Wynder EL, Mabuchi K, Beattie EJ: The epidemiology of
   lung cancer. Recent trends. JAMA 213: 2221-2228, 1970.
2. Yesner R, Gelfman NA, Feinstein AR: A reappraisal of
   histopathology of lung cancer and correlation of cell type
   with antecedent cigarette smoking. Amer Rev Resp Dis 107:
   790-797, 1973.
3. Scherrer M, Zeller CH, Christen H, Bachofen H, Senn A,
   Zimmermann H: Der Lungenkrebs in der Region Bern. Schweiz
   med Wschr 106: 1167-1173, 1976.
4. Mcd. Herrold K: Survey of histologic types of primary
   lung cancer in U.S. veterans.
   Path Ann 7: 45-79, 1972.
5. Larsson S: Completeness and reliability of lung cancer
   registration in the Swedish cancer registry. Acta path
   microbiol scand. Sect. A 79: 389-398, 1971.
6. Petersen GF: Incidence of pulmonary carcinoma in Iceland
   between 1931 and 1964. Acta Radiologica 11: 321-326, 1972.
7. Chan WC, Colbourne MJ, Fung SC, Ho HC: Bronchial cancer in
   Hong Kong 1976-1977. Br J Cancer 39: 182, 1979.
8. Kung ITM, So KF, Lam TH: Lung cancer in Hong Kong Chinese:
   Mortality and histological types, 1973-1982. Brit J Cancer
   50: 381-388, 1984.
9. Reinila A, Dammert K: An attempt to use the WHO typing
   in the histological classification of lung carcinomas.
   Acta path microbiol scand. Sect. A 82: 783-790, 1974.
10. Vincent RG, Pickren JW, Lane WW, Bross I, Takita H,
    Houten L, Gutierrez AC, Rzepka T: The changing histo
    pathology of lung cancer. Cancer 39: 1647-1655, 1977.

FIGURE 1.

Correlation of cigarette consumption
and histological cell type (WHO)

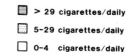

- ▦ > 29 cigarettes/daily
- ▨ 5-29 cigarettes/daily
- ☐ 0-4 cigarettes/daily

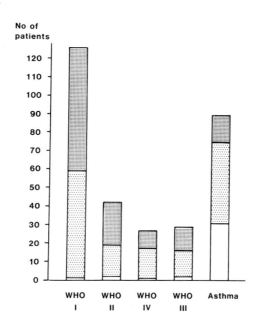

TABLE 1.

Comparison of histological types by classification according to WHO recommendations (1967) and types recorded in the Cancer Registry (5).

	Cancer Registry		WHO-recommendations		
	No.	%	I	II+IV	III
Epidermoid	224	41.5	77.2	13.0	9.4
Anaplastic	234	43.0	32.9	46.0	16.7
Adenocarcinoma	64	12.0	3.0	11.0	78.8

TABLE 2.

Distribution by cell type (%).
1967 WHO classification.

	N*	WHO I	II	III	IV	(ref.)
Bern 1974-76	223	56.0	19.0	13.0	12.0	3
Iceland 1931-64	136	17.4	33.6	22.8	16.8	6
Hong Kong 1960-72	853	36.8	22.2	21.6	15.8	7
Hong Kong 1973-82	1055	30.7	19.1	36.4	13.8	8
Finland 1968-71	175	54.2	29.7	8.6	0.6	9

N: number of patients

TABLE 3.

Percentage distribution of histological types
(WHO 1967) in 2 series of lung cancer in
Hong Kong (8).

Histological types

Period	I ♂	I ♀	II ♂	II ♀	III ♂	III ♀	IV ♂	IV ♀	Others ♂	Others ♀
1960-1972*	43.6	22.7	21.5	23.8	15.6	34.3	15.8	16.2	3.5	2.9
1973-1982**	33.3	22.6	21.3	12.6	25.8	49.6	14.7	10.6	4.7	5.3

* : includes 576 males, 277 females
**: includes 714 males, 341 females

TABLE 4.

Percentage distribution of histological types of
lung cancer in University Department of Pathology
Hong Kong Island 1979-1982 (8).

A comparison of 1967 and 1981 classification

	WHO 1967	WHO 1981
WHO I	29.7	29.7
WHO II	19.1	19.1
WHO III	33.2	40.3
WHO IV	13.1	6.0
Others	4.9	4.9

SQUAMOUS CELL CARCINOMA AND UNDIFFERENTIATED LARGE CELL CARCINOMA OF LUNG:
SIMILARITIES AND DIFFERENCES

L.B. WOOLNER

1. INTRODUCTION

Primary lung cancer is currently categorized into four histologic
subtypes according to the World Health Organization Histological Typing of
Lung Tumours.[1] These subtypes are squamous cell carcinoma, small cell
carcinoma, adenocarcinoma, and large cell carcinoma. Each of these
subtypes is, in turn, subdivided into one or more variants; combined forms
also occur. The criteria for diagnosis are based on light microscopic
observations only.

The classification of the World Health Organization has proved relatively
satisfactory for pathologists. The category that provides the most
diagnostic difficulty is large cell carcinoma, which is defined as lacking
the characteristic features of squamous cell carcinoma, small cell
carcinoma, or adenocarcinoma. Unfortunately, very poorly differentiated
squamous cell carcinoma or adenocarcinoma is difficult to distinguish
clearly from "undifferentiated" cancer. Obviously, any highly malignant
carcinoma of nonsmall cell type with equivocal or borderline evidence of
differentiation may present difficulties with respect to diagnostic
reproducibility; the most reproducible results seem to be favored by
diagnosing large cell carcinoma in cases of this sort. Other diagnostic
difficulties may occur with completely undifferentiated carcinomas whose
nuclei are "intermediate" as opposed to being small or large; also, the
precise definition of bronchiolo-alveolar carcinoma within the confines of
the adenocarcinoma subgroup is unclear.

Some differences in the biologic behavior or in the clinicopathologic
manifestations are observed among the four subgroups of lung cancer, and
certain general concepts have been widely accepted regarding the individual
cell types. Thus, squamous cell carcinoma is frequently described as being
the most common, predominantly intrabronchial in origin, largely central
in location, and relatively less aggressive and as having a more favorable
prognosis. Small cell carcinoma is primarily central in origin, is
characterized by rapid growth and dissemination, and is associated with a
uniformly fatal outcome. Large cell carcinoma and adenocarcinoma have
several manifestations in common, including a peripheral location, fairly
rapid dissemination, and a prognosis midway between that associated with
squamous cell and small cell carcinoma.

Small cell carcinoma is generally agreed to differ so significantly from
the other cell types in biologic behavior and response to therapy that it
must be considered a separate entity with regard to classification and
treatment. The usefulness of dividing nonsmall cell carcinoma into
distinct entities may be questionable, particularly with regard to
long-term prognosis.

The purpose of this chapter is to examine some of the similarities and
differences among the three nonsmall cell types of lung cancer, especially

the squamous cell and large cell types. The salient features (relative frequency, site of origin, gross and microscopic pathologic features, aggressiveness, staging, and prognosis) of each of the three subtypes are summarized.

The data are based on studies of 1) surgically resected lung cancers found in ordinary clinical practice at the Mayo Clinic (primarily surgical series) and 2) lung cancers diagnosed during the course of screening a high-risk population of Mayo Clinic patients for early lung cancer. When possible, the data from these two sources are compared with data from the recent literature.

The screening study (Mayo Lung Project) involved an initial prevalence screening of high-risk subjects and their subsequent randomization into a close surveillance (screening every 4 months) group and a comparison (control) group. A total of 206 "incidence" cancers were detected in the close surveillance group up to July 1, 1983, and 160 incidence cancers were detected in the control group during the same period. Details of the protocol and findings of the Mayo Lung Project have been published.[2-6]

2. RELATIVE FREQUENCY OF CELL TYPES

Misleading impressions about the relative frequency of the subtypes of lung cancer may be derived from surgical series in which the number of each subtype depends on operability. Similarly, prevalence screening may provide biased estimates; slowly growing tumors, detectable over a long time, tend to be oversampled, and rapidly growing cancers, detectable for a short period, tend to be undersampled. The relative frequencies of each cell type in male cigarette smokers according to prevalence and incidence screening in the Mayo Lung Project through December 1979 are compared in Table 1.[4,5] The true relative frequency of squamous cell carcinoma in the incidence screening was 30% (a decrease from 43% in the prevalence screening). Similarly, the true relative frequency of small cell carcinoma in the incidence screening was 26% (an increase from 13% in the prevalence screening). Large cell carcinoma (19% in the incidence screening) was the least common subtype. This finding is common to that of most published series, but, as indicated above, the exact relative frequency of large cell carcinoma is uniquely dependent on the histologic criteria used by the pathologist to define the three other subtypes.

TABLE 1. Frequencies of subtypes of lung cancer according to prevalence and incidence screening in the Mayo Lung Project

Cell type	Prevalence (N = 91)		Incidence (N = 109)*	
	No. pt	%	No. pt	%
Squamous	39	43	33	30
Adenocarcinoma	25	27	26	24
Large	15	17	21	19
Small	12	13	28	26
Bronchial carcinoid	...	...	1	1
Total	91	100	109	100

*Includes 18 "dropout" cases (cases in which cancer developed at some time after patient withdrew from the screening program).
From Woolner et al.[5] By permission of Mayo Foundation.

The percentages of the relative frequencies for the squamous cell and
small cell subtypes are in sharp contrast to those reported in many
surgical series or prevalence studies, in which the relative frequency of
squamous cell carcinoma is 40% to 55% and that of small cell carcinoma is
5% to 10%.

In addition to the histologic criteria used for diagnosis, the relative
frequencies of the cell types of lung cancer depend on additional factors
such as the sex ratio of the patients being studied as well as occupational
exposure and geographic location. In several recent studies, the relative
proportion of adenocarcinoma seemed to be increasing.[7,8]

3. PATHOLOGY

3.1. Microscopic variants of squamous cell and large cell carcinoma

Squamous cell carcinoma, as defined in the classification of the World
Health Organization, may be well differentiated, moderately differentiated,
or poorly differentiated. Extremely well-differentiated squamous cell carcinoma (Fig. 1a) is uncommon in the lung, moderately differentiated tumors
(Fig. 1b) are common, and poorly differentiated tumors (Fig. 1c) account
for most cases. In a series of 252 resected squamous cell carcinomas
reviewed by the author,[9] 5 (2%) were well differentiated, 93 (37%) were
moderately differentiated, and 154 (61%) were poorly differentiated. The
poorly differentiated tumors merge imperceptibly into the category of large
cell undifferentiated carcinoma, as discussed above. Occult (sputum-
positive, roentgenogram-negative) carcinomas (see below), which are almost
invariably the squamous cell type, may be well or poorly differentiated,
but most have a moderate degree of squamatization and maturation.[6]

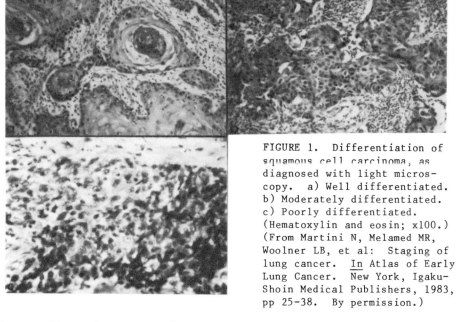

FIGURE 1. Differentiation of
squamous cell carcinoma, as
diagnosed with light microscopy. a) Well differentiated.
b) Moderately differentiated.
c) Poorly differentiated.
(Hematoxylin and eosin; x100.)
(From Martini N, Melamed MR,
Woolner LB, et al: Staging of
lung cancer. In Atlas of Early
Lung Cancer. New York, Igaku-
Shoin Medical Publishers, 1983,
pp 25-38. By permission.)

Large cell carcinoma, a malignant tumor with large nuclei, is one that
lacks the characteristic features of squamous cell carcinoma,

adenocarcinoma, or small cell carcinoma when viewed with light microscopy. Ultrastructural studies, however, have shown that many tumors that are categorized as large cell carcinomas may have some evidence of adenocarcinoma or squamous cell differentiation or both.[10] Classic examples of these highly anaplastic carcinomas are shown in Figure 2. Rather uncommon variants include giant cell carcinoma (Fig. 3a) and clear cell carcinoma (Fig. 3b). In a series of 160 surgically resected large cell carcinomas reviewed by the author, giant cell and clear cell variants accounted for 8% and 5%, respectively, of the total.[9]

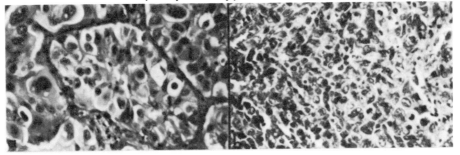

FIGURE 2. Large cell carcinoma. a) Large cells with abundant cytoplasm. b) Undifferentiated growth pattern with numerous mitotic figures. (Hematoxylin and eosin; x250.) (From Martini N, Melamed MR, Woolner LB, et al: Staging of lung cancer. In Atlas of Early Lung Cancer. New York, Igaku-Shoin Medical Publishers, 1983, pp 25-38. By permission.)

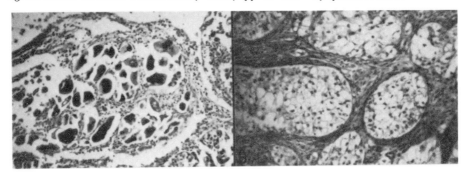

FIGURE 3. Variants of large cell carcinoma. a) Giant cell variant. b) Clear cell variant. (Hematoxylin and eosin; x100.) (From Martini N, Melamed MR, Woolner LB, et al: Staging of lung cancer. In Atlas of Early Lung Cancer. New York, Igaku-Shoin Medical Publishers, 1983, pp 25-38. By permission.)

3.2 Site of origin

Primary lung cancers may arise from any portion of the bronchial epithelial lining from the carina to the region of the pleura and, therefore, may be classified as "central" or "peripheral." As defined by a pathologist or bronchoscopist, a central carcinoma is one involving subsegmental or more proximal bronchi, and a peripheral tumor is one that occurs more distally within the parenchyma all the way to the pleura.

Central tumors may thus be readily seen or brushed by a bronchoscopist, and peripheral tumors are less accessible with this approach.

A radiologist may classify a tumor as central if it is located at the hilus or within 4 cm of the hilus and as peripheral if it is more than 4 cm from the hilus.[11] The site of origin of a lung tumor, whether from a large bronchus or from lung parenchyma, has considerable bearing on features such as clinical presentation, gross morphologic findings, and methods of diagnosis.

Squamous cell carcinoma may arise anywhere from the main carina to the pleura; thus, it may be central or peripheral. Many squamous cell carcinomas arise from the large bronchi (segmental or more proximal) and, by intrabronchial and extrabronchial extension, form a characteristic polypoid and infiltrative mass that eventually surrounds and obstructs the involved bronchial segment. Gross variants that involve large bronchi have been classified as polypoid, nodular infiltrating, or superficial infiltrating.[12]

Occult lung carcinomas (that is, sputum-positive, roentgenogram-negative) are central squamous cell carcinomas. In the Mayo Lung Project,[6] the exact sites of origin and gross and microscopic findings were determined for 68 such carcinomas, all of which were surgically resected and subjected to extensive serial block sectioning. The segmental bronchi with or without involvement of the lobar bronchi were by far the most frequent sites of origin of these very early squamous cell carcinomas. In addition to the small, rather localized examples, very widespread carcinomatous involvement of the bronchial mucosa from the main bronchus to the segmental bronchi was occasionally encountered (Table 2).

TABLE 2. Sites of origin of 68 occult lung carcinomas in the Mayo Lung Project (November 1971 through December 1981)

Site (bronchus)	No. of cases (%)
Main	3 (4.0)
Main and lobar	1 (1.5)
Main, lobar, and segmental	3 (4.0)
Lobar	2 (3.0)
Lobar and segmental	23 (34)
Segmental	35 (51)
Subsegmental	1 (1.5)
Total	68 100

Somewhat less anatomically precise information about the location of lung cancers by cell type is provided by roentgenographic studies. The roentgenographic findings in a large series of lung cancers diagnosed in a clinical setting and classified according to cell type were reported by Byrd et al.[13] In their study, 40% of squamous cell carcinomas manifested as a hilar or perihilar mass. In the Mayo Lung Project, a series of 92 roentgenographically visible incidence lung cancers detected through roentgenographic screening every 4 months was described by Muhm et al.[11] At the time of detection, more than 50% of these cancers were classified as stage I according to the system of the American Joint Committee on Cancer (AJCC).[14] Squamous cell carcinomas were almost equally distributed between central and peripheral locations. By contrast, most large cell carcinomas (and adenocarcinomas) were peripheral (Table 3).

The distribution of 206 lung cancers, the total number of incidence lung cancers detected in the close surveillance (screening every 4 months) group of the Mayo Lung Project, was studied by Fontana.[15] The series included occult as well as roentgenogram-positive cancers, and the classification (central or peripheral) was based on all available evidence, including roentgenographic, pathologic, and bronchoscopic data. This particular classification is subject to some inaccuracy in that large tumors that were visible bronchoscopically may have arisen in a peripheral location and extended centrally into a bronchus. This combined approach to classification was used to determine the locations for each cell type (Table 4).

TABLE 3. Cell type and location of 92 roentgenographically visible incidence lung cancers in the Mayo Lung Project diagnosed up to January 1982

	Location, no. pt				
		Central			
Cell type	Periph-eral	Peri-hilar	Hilar enlargement or paratracheal adenopathy	Pneumo-nitis	Total
Squamous	12	6	6	1	25
Adenocarcinoma	18	1	2	1	22
Large	11	1	1	1	14
Small	6	8	11	2	27
Alveolar	2	0	0	0	2
Mixed squamous and large	1	0	0	0	1
Carcinoid	...	0	0	1	1
	50	16	20	6	92

From Muhm et al.[11] By permission of the Radiological Society of North America.

TABLE 4. Cell type and location of 206 incidence lung cancers in the Mayo Lung Project detected from November 1971 through July 1, 1983

	Location, %	
Cell type, no. cases	Central	Peripheral
Squamous, 68	45	55
Adenocarcinoma, 61	20	80
Large cell, 29	33	67
Small cell, 48	75	25

3.3 Gross morphologic findings

Peripheral lung cancers, as defined, may be of any cell type; however, the most common type is adenocarcinoma. The peripherally placed carcinomas have somewhat less varied gross morphologic features than the more centrally placed tumors. They generally manifest during the early stage of development as small, rounded parenchymal nodules ("coin lesions") and as larger, fairly sharply circumscribed masses during the later stages. The smallest lesions detected roentgenographically are about 1.0 cm in diameter,[11] the approximate lower limit of detectability. The cut surface of a peripheral lesion is unlikely to be diagnostic for cell type, but some differences in the gross morphologic features of each type may be noted (Fig. 4). Squamous cell carcinomas are likely to demonstrate gross bronchial communication and thus are the most likely to have positive cytologic findings. Large squamous cell carcinomas are the most likely to undergo central necrosis and cavitation and also are generally associated with positive cytologic findings. Central fibrosis and anthracosis may occur in a peripheral cancer of any cell type (except small cell) but are more characteristic of adenocarcinoma.[16] Associated pleural indentation and puckering are also highly characteristic of adenocarcinoma, but they may occur with other nonsmall cell types. Rapidly growing large cell peripheral carcinomas may be softer and less likely to exhibit puckering of the overlying pleura.

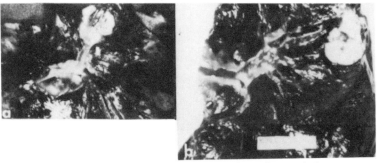

FIGURE 4. Gross morphologic features of peripheral lung cancer.
a) Subpleural squamous cell carcinoma showing bronchial communication.
b) Large cell carcinoma not obviously related to a bronchus.

4. AGGRESSIVENESS AND STAGING

Not all lung cancers progress at the same rate. The speed of dissemination of the various subtypes has an obvious bearing on the type of treatment and prognosis. A measure of the extent of disease at any given time is best provided by the TNM staging system, as outlined by the AJCC.[14]

Small cell carcinoma grows and disseminates rapidly. In clinical practice (and even in a close-surveillance screening project), most cases are detected at clinical stage III of the AJCC. AJCC staging is of little practical value for the determination of treatment and prognosis for patients with this type of tumor.

Occult (sputum-positive, roentgenogram-negative) carcinomas, a relatively small group of central squamous cell cancers that are detected through screening, appear to evolve slowly through in situ, microinvasive, and more deeply invasive stages. In a series of 68 surgically resected cases, a third of the tumors were in situ, a third were microinvasive, and a third were deeply invasive into or through the bronchial wall.[6]

AJCC staging at the time of diagnosis may be used to compare progression of cancer in the various nonsmall cell subtypes. Data on 206 incidence cancers, the total number of cases in the close surveillance (screening every 4 months) group in the Mayo Lung Project, are shown in Table 5.[14] Each of the nonsmall cell subtypes had a proportion of carcinomas detected

in postsurgical resection-pathologic stage I or II (resectable stage).
However, each category also had a surprisingly large number of stage III
and unresectable cancers. When the roentgenographically "occult"
carcinomas are excluded, approximately 44% of each nonsmall cell subtype
was classified as postsurgical stages I or II and 56% as stage III at the
time of diagnosis.

Roentgenographic data illustrating two rates of tumor progression were
presented by Muhm et al.[11] In the 92 cases of roentgenographically visible
incidence lung cancers referred to above (Table 3), serial chest
roentgenograms obtained every 4 months showed that a surprising number of
carcinomas were visible in retrospect after the initial roentgenographic
diagnosis. The two growth patterns described by Muhm were 1) slowly
growing peripheral or perihilar nodules usually visible in retrospect after
they had been detected initially and 2) central cancers that grew rapidly
and seemed to "explode" and cause considerable enlargement of the hilus or
mediastinal structures after a recent roentgenographic examination of the
chest showed normal findings.

TABLE 5. Staging at time of diagnosis for 206 incidence lung cancers in
the Mayo Lung Project detected from November 1971 through July 1, 1983

Stage	Cell type, no. cases				
	Squamous	Adenocarcinoma	Large	Small	Total
Postsurgical resection-pathologic stage I	35*	25	12	6	78
Postsurgical resection-pathologic stage II	3†	1	1†		5
Stage III and unresectable	30	35	16	42	123
Total	68	61	29	48	206

*Includes 14 cases detected cytologically.
†Includes one case detected cytologically.

5. PROGNOSIS

Data on the prognosis of patients with lung cancer according to the AJCC
stage at the time of diagnosis and according to cell type can be derived
from surgical series, cases detected through prevalence screening, or
incidence cases detected in screening programs such as the Mayo Lung
Project. The prognosis after treatment seems to be uniformly hopeless for
patients with small cell cancer and somewhat more encouraging for those
with the three other cell types. The most important determinant of
prognosis for patients with the nonsmall cell types is the postsurgical
resection-pathologic stage (AJCC) at the time of diagnosis. The 5-year
survival after surgical treatment for patients with postsurgical resection-
pathologic stage I nonsmall cell cancer has been reported to be close to
70%, and that for stage III (and unresectable) cancer is less than 10%.

A review of the recent literature in an attempt to compare the results of
surgical treatment for the three nonsmall cell types reveals a surprising
degree of uniformity in most reported series of "clinical practice" cases.
Thus, Williams and associates[17] reported an overall 5-year survival of 69%
for a Mayo Clinic series of 495 patients with surgical-postsurgical AJCC
stage I lung cancers (from 1972-1978) and no overall significant difference
in survival on the basis of cell type (the 5-year survival was 70% for

patients with squamous cell cancer, 65% for those with adenocarcinoma, and 66% for those with large cell carcinoma). Kemeny et al. and Martini et al. also reported comparably high 5-year survival rates for patients with postsurgical stage I nonsmall cell cancers[18] and a 5-year survival rate of 29% for patients with more advanced disease and mediastinal lymph node metastasis (N2--that is, patients who had complete, potentially curable resection of the primary tumor and all accessible mediastinal lymph nodes).[19] Neither category had a difference in survival rates among the cases of nonsmall cell types. Mountain[20] reported no essential differences in the 5-year survival rate for patients with postsurgical stage I squamous cell cancer and a combined group of patients with adenocarcinoma or large cell carcinoma--the approximate rate for those with squamous cell carcinoma was 56% and that for the combined group was 53%.

Similarly, in a prior Mayo Clinic series of surgically resected cases (unstaged), Galofré et al.[21] reported 10-year survival rates that were approximately equal for patients with squamous cell and large cell carcinoma and slightly lower for those with adenocarcinoma. Shields et al.,[22] in a large series of treated lung cancers (unstaged but classified as to presence or absence of metastatic lymph nodes), found no significant differences in 5-year or 10-year survival among the three nonsmall cell types. The survival data reported by Vincent et al.[23] for 295 surgically resected cases that were studied between 1963 and 1974 were not significantly different among the three nonsmall cell types.

The survival data for all incidence cancers in the Mayo Lung Project, except those detected cytologically, support the aforementioned clinical studies.[15] Survival curves according to the various cell types of the incidence cancers show that the survival rates for nonoccult, postsurgical stage I and II (AJCC) lung cancers of the three nonsmall cell types are similar (Fig. 5), as are the survival rates for stage III (and unresectable) cancers of all four cell types (Fig. 6). The 5-year survival for patients with stage I or II squamous cell carcinoma, adenocarcinoma, and large cell carcinoma averaged 50% to 60% and that for patients with small cell carcinoma was less than 15%. The 5-year survival for patients with stage III and unresectable cancers of all four cell types was less than 10%.

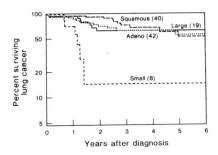

FIGURE 5. Survival rates for 109 postsurgical stage I and II (AJCC) incidence cases of lung cancer detected in Mayo Lung Project (excludes cases detected cytologically).

6. DISCUSSION

Pathologic studies of "surgical series" of lung cancer provide much useful information about the sites of origin, gross morphologic findings, and the extent of spread. Such studies are essential, but the data obtained in these studies provide information about only that proportion of lung carcinoma that is surgically resected. Comprehensive screening studies of lung cancer, such as that outlined above, provide data about both operable and inoperable cases, give more reliable information about the relative frequency of types of cancer, and reflect a more balanced view of lung cancer as a whole.

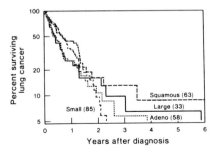

FIGURE 6. Survival rates for 239 stage III (AJCC) and unresectable incidence cases of lung cancer detected in Mayo Lung Project from November 1971 to July 1983 (excludes cases detected cytologically).

Data from incidence screening studies indicate that squamous cell carcinoma is not as common as suggested by many reported surgical series. Squamous cell carcinomas accounted for only a third of all lung cancer in male cigarette smokers in recently completed screening studies. The frequency of occult carcinoma, a special subcategory of squamous cell carcinoma, has long been a subject for speculation. Incidence screening determined that this sputum-positive, roentgenogram-negative component of lung cancer is not common—it accounted for about 10% to 15% of all lung cancers in the Mayo Lung Project.[5] This finding was a major disappointment in the screening program because a much larger proportion of such early, potentially curable squamous cell carcinomas was anticipated.

Large cell carcinoma is less frequently diagnosed than squamous cell carcinoma, and its exact relative frequency will vary somewhat according to the definition used. Reproducible results are favored by categorizing all cases with equivocal evidence of squamous cell carcinoma or adenocarcinoma differentiation as large cell carcinoma. With the use of these criteria, large cell carcinoma will not constitute more than 15% to 20% of all lung cancers (this percentage will be much lower if other histologic definitions are used).

The site of origin for lung cancer is readily determined for stage I and II (AJCC) surgically resected cases; the site is much more difficult to determine for cases of advanced carcinoma. Certain bulky, surgically resected cancers may extend from the hilus almost to the pleura; thus, the exact point of origin will be questionable. Stage III (AJCC) and unresectable cases are generally also difficult to classify as to location (central or peripheral). The approach used in the screening study for all incidence cases in the Mayo Lung Project (Table 4) provides the most accurate approximation of location, but the fact that some peripheral cancers may extend centrally and involve larger bronchi must be kept in mind. Adenocarcinoma and small cell carcinoma provide the sharpest contrast as to site of origin. Adenocarcinoma seldom involves large central bronchi and is predominantly parenchymal and subpleural. Small cell carcinoma is largely central, and only a few cases manifest as peripheral nodules. The contrast between squamous cell and large cell carcinoma is less pronounced, but the latter demonstrates a somewhat greater propensity for a peripheral location. Occult carcinomas are almost always central and squamous, although rare mixed squamous and large cell examples have been described.

All evidence points to a remarkable similarity in aggressiveness among the three nonsmall cell subtypes of lung cancer, as judged by AJCC staging of cases detected in a population undergoing surveillance in a screening program. The percentage of each subtype detected at combined AJCC stages I and II was approximately 44%. This calculation excludes occult squamous cell carcinoma, a small subgroup that is unlikely to be detected in the absence of a cytologic screening program.

Roentgenographic studies of incidence cancers in a screening program described by Muhm et al.[11] showed that "visibility in retrospect" is present for a surprising number of incidence carcinomas in all three nonsmall cell types. This finding is particularly marked for peripheral or perihilar nodules, in which prior roentgenograms often show an undetected small lesion for 2 years or more. Unfortunately, no test or procedure is currently available to determine the potential for dissemination for any single nonsmall cell cancer--one knows only that some of these tumors can remain relatively quiescent for rather long periods and others will spread rapidly.

7. CONCLUSIONS

A comparison of the cell types of lung cancer that uses data from "clinical practice" sources and from recent screening studies for early lung cancer points to the following general conclusions.

In all important respects, small cell carcinoma is sufficiently different from nonsmall cell carcinoma that it should be considered a separate entity in any scheme of classification or in treatment protocols. Nonsmall cell carcinomas have major histologic differences and some differences in clinical presentation and the approach to bronchoscopic or cytologic diagnosis. However, these differences seem rather unimportant when the three cell types are compared in the larger context of staging (AJCC), treatment, and prognosis; thus, all three nonsmall cell types might be combined for such essential considerations. Instead of more detailed comparisons of the cell types, attention might better be focused on a comparison of the "early," resectable (and perhaps potentially curable) component of nonsmall cell carcinoma with the "late," generally unresectable component. Efforts to explain the basic differences in the aggressiveness between these two "subgroups" (that is, stage I [AJCC] and stage III [AJCC] and unresectable types) seem to hold more promise than a continued comparison of the three nonsmall cell subtypes.

REFERENCES

1. World Health Organization: The World Health Organization histological typing of lung tumours. Second edition. Am J Clin Pathol 77:123-136, 1982.
2. Fontana RS, Sanderson DR, Miller WE, et al: The Mayo Lung Project: preliminary report of "early cancer detection" phase. Cancer 30: 1373-1382, 1972.
3. Fontana RS, Sanderson DR, Woolner LB, et al: The Mayo Lung Project for early detection and localization of bronchogenic carcinoma: a status report. Chest 67:511-522, 1975.
4. Fontana RS, Sanderson DR, Taylor WF, et al: Early lung cancer detection: results of the initial (prevalence) radiologic and cytologic screening in the Mayo Clinic study. Am Rev Respir Dis 130: 561-565, 1984.

5. Woolner LB, Fontana RS, Sanderson DR, et al: Mayo Lung Project: evaluation of lung cancer screening through December 1979. Mayo Clin Proc 56:544-555, 1981.
6. Woolner LB, Fontana RS, Cortese DA, et al: Roentgenographically occult lung cancer: pathologic findings and frequency of multi-centricity during a 10-year period. Mayo Clin Proc 59:453-466, 1984.
7. Vincent RG, Pickren JW, Lane WW, et al: The changing histopathology of lung cancer: a review of 1682 cases. Cancer 39:1647-1655, 1977.
8. Melamed MR, Flehinger BJ, Zaman MB, et al: Screening for early lung cancer: results of the Memorial Sloan-Kettering Study in New York. Chest 86:44-53, 1984.
9. Woolner LB: Unpublished data.
10. Horie A, Ohta M: Ultrastructural features of large cell carcinoma of the lung with reference to the prognosis of patients. Hum Pathol 12: 423-432, 1981.
11. Muhm JR, Miller WE, Fontana RS, et al: Lung cancer detected during a screening program using four-month chest radiographs. Radiology 148: 609-615, 1983.
12. Shimosato Y: Pathology of lung cancer. Excerpta Medica International Congress Series No 525, 1980, pp 27-48.
13. Byrd RB, Carr DT, Miller WE, et al: Radiographic abnormalities in carcinoma of the lung as related to histological cell type. Thorax 24:573-575, 1969.
14. American Joint Committee on Cancer: Manual for Staging of Cancer. Second edition. Edited by OH Beahrs, MH Myers. Philadelphia, JB Lippincott Company, 1983, pp 99-105.
15. Fontana RS: Unpublished data.
16. Shimosato Y, Hashimoto T, Kodama T, et al: Prognostic implications of fibrotic focus (scar) in small peripheral lung cancers. Am J Surg Pathol 4:365-373, 1980.
17. Williams DE, Pairolero PC, Davis CS, et al: Survival of patients surgically treated for Stage I lung cancer. J Thorac Cardiovasc Surg 82:70-76, 1981.
18. Kemeny MM, Block LR, Braun DW Jr, et al: Results of surgical treat-ment of carcinoma of the lung by stage and cell type. Surg Gynecol Obstet 147:865-871, 1978.
19. Martini N, Flehinger BJ, Zaman MB, et al: Results of resection in non-oat cell carcinoma of the lung with mediastinal lymph node metastases. Ann Surg 198:386-396, 1983.
20. American Joint Committee for Cancer Staging and End-Results Reporting and Task Force on Lung: Staging of Lung Cancer. 1979, 24 pp. Published by the American Joint Committee, 55 East Erie Street, Chicago IL 60611.
21. Galofré M, Payne WS, Woolner LB, et al: Pathologic classification and surgical treatment of bronchogenic carcinoma. Surg Gynecol Obstet 119:51-61, 1964.
22. Shields TW, Yee J, Conn JH, et al: Relationship of cell type and lymph node metastasis to survival after resection of bronchial carcinoma. Ann Thorac Surg 20:501-510, 1975.
23. Vincent RG, Takita H, Lane WW, et al: Surgical therapy of lung cancer. J Thorac Cardiovasc Surg 71:581-591, 1976.

ADENOCARCINOMA: CLINICAL SIGNIFICANCE OF SUBTYPING AND OTHER MORPHOLOGIC FACTORS

YUKIO SHIMOSATO and TETSURO KODAMA

1.INTRODUCTION
Adenocarcinoma is the most frequent lung cancer in Japan as well as in some other oriental countries. It accounted for 46.5% of 1209 surgically resected lung cancers and 44.3% of 879 autopsied lung cancers during the period of 1962 through 1981 at the National Cancer Center Hospital (1).

The actual 5-year survival rate of resected adenocarcinoma cases was 26.8% and that in Stage Ia was 63.0% (unpublished data). Of course, the most significant and prevalently used prognostic factors are T, N and M factors. Accordingly pleural involvement, lymph node metastasis and distant organ metastasis are the most important and easily recognized pathological parameters. However, there are many other morphological factors, which are thought to affect prognosis. These include histologic and cytologic subtypes, degrees of differentiation and cell atypia, cell kinetics, vascular invasion, host response, etc. In this chapter, the cytologic subtyping of adenocarcinoma, presently used in Japan (1, 2, 3), is described and the relationship between those morphologic factors seen in surgically resected materials and 5-year survival rate is dealt with.

2.MATERIALS AND METHODS
Among 675 surgically resected adenocarcinoma cases during the period from 1962 through 1983, 85 cases evaluable for 5 years after surgery with a tumor less than 3 cm in diameter and 75 cases with tumors less than 2 cm were analyzed in terms of the morphologic factors and survival of patients. Follow up data were available in all cases.

Histologic sections, including at least the largest cut surface of tumors, were stained routinely with hematoxylin and eosin and elastica stain. For electron microscopy, minced tissues were routinely processed and embedded in Epon 812. Ultrathin sections were examined with a JEOL 100U electron microscope after staining with uranium and lead. For immunohistochemistry, peroxidase-antiperoxidase complex or avidin-biotin-peroxidase complex method was employed using antibodies to secretory component, lactoferrin, S100 protein (DAKO, Copenhagen, Denmark), and surfactant apoprotein (a gift of Dr. G. Singh, Department of Pathology, University of Pittsburgh, U.S.A.) and monoclonal antibody OKT 6 (Ortho Pharmaceutical, U.S.A.). The nuclear area and its standard deviation were calculated by an image analyzer (Kontron MOP-AMO3).

The actual 5-year survival rate was obtained for cases with tumors less than 3 cm in diameter, all of which were resected at least 5 years ago. Statistical significance was analyzed by the chi-square test. Separately, for cases with a tumor less than 2 cm in diameter, survival curves were obtained by the Kaplan-Meier method and prognostic factors were analyzed by Peto's logrank test.

3.SUBTYPING: HISTOLOGIC AND CYTOLOGIC

Adenocarcinoma has been subdivided histologically by the WHO classification into acinar, papillary, bronchioloalveolar and solid tumor with mucus formation. It is also subdivided by the degree of differentiation into well, moderately and poorly differentiated tumor (4). However, some of those histologic subtypes, particularly papillary and bronchioloalveolar types, consist of a variety of tumors from the cytological view point. Therefore, it is important to classify the tumor not only from the histological structure but also from the cytological characteristics, i.e. the direction of cell differentiation, in order to understand the biology of a given tumor and to predict prognosis.

The direction of cell differentiation can be suspected not only by routine histology and histochemistry and electron-microscopy, but also by the recently developed immunohistochemical method to detect antigenic substances specific to certain cell type in the airway. From our experience many adenocarcinomas of less than 1.5 cm in diameter are composed of tumor cells of a single cell type. As the tumor becomes larger, the frequency of and areas occupied by metaplastic tumor cells become larger, which complicates the biology of tumors. The term metaplasia used here means appearance of tumor cells differentiating toward a different direction from the original tumor cells, i.e. from Clara cell to mucus producing cells.

Adenocarcinoma cells are supposed to differentiate toward either one of the following cell types; ciliated columnar cells, goblet cells, intermediate or indifferent cells, Clara cells, type II (or perhaps type I) alveolar epithelial cells, bronchial gland duct cells, mucus cells, serous cells, myoepithelial cells, etc. For the sake of convenience, we subclassify adenocarcinoma of the lung into following 6 cytological types (3).
a. bronchial surface cell type with little or no mucus production
b. goblet cell type
c. bronchial gland cell type
d. Clara cell type
e. type II alveolar epithelial cell type
f. mixed cell type

3.1.Bronchial surface cell type with little or no mucus production

Tumor cells are tall and columnar with basal or irregularly dispersed nuclei, arranged frequently in a papillary fashion.

No cilia can be seen. The secretory component can frequently

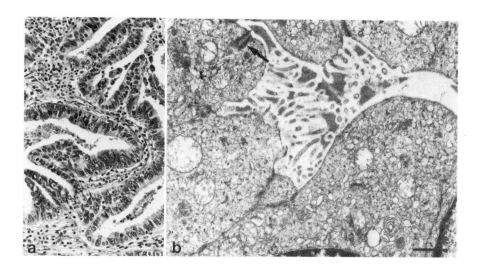

FIGURE 1. a) Histology of bronchial surface epithelial cell
type reveals tall columnar cells arranged in a papillary
pattern. b) Ultrastructurally they possess many smooth
surfaced vesicles, occasional mitochondria, basal body (arrow)
and microvilli.

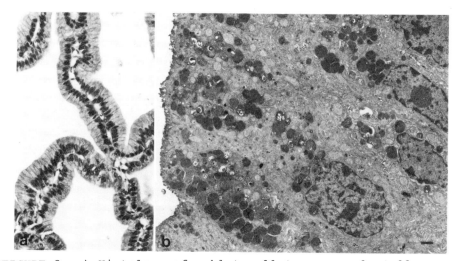

FIGURE 2. a) Histology of goblet cell type reveals tall
columnar cells with basal nuclei, which replace the alveolar
lining cells. b) Ultrastructurally cytoplasm is filled with
mucus granules.

be detected immunohistochemically. Ultrastructurally, they
are rich in mitochondria and small smooth surfaced vesicles
but with few, if any, secretory granules. Basal bodies are
frequent at the free cell border, indicating that the cells
differentiate toward ciliated cells (Fig. 1). The tumor
originates in both cartilage bearing and more peripheral
bronchi. Endobronchial polypoid growth may be seen (5, 6).
This type of adenocarcinoma was seen in about 8% of our
materials.

3.2. Goblet cell type

Tumor cells with abundant cytoplasmic mucin and basal nuclei
resemble goblet cells, and are arranged in a
bronchioloalveolar or papillary pattern. Ultrastructurally,
mucus granules filling the cytoplasm generally show low
electron density and variable internal structures (Fig. 2) (2,
3, 7). Immunostain for lactoferrin is negative. Tumors of
this type are relatively infrequent. "Alveolar cell carcinoma
of lobar distribution" is a typical representative case.

3.3. Bronchial gland cell type

Cuboidal cells are arranged in acinar, tubular or cribriform
patterns and frequently produce mucin. Mucin-containing
signet ring cells may form solid nests. Electron
microscopically, mucus granules of varying electron density
and rather characteristic fibrillar inclusions are seen (Fig.
3). Granules suggestive of duct type or serous type may be
seen. At the border of cell nests, cells resembling
myoepithelial cells with myofibril-like fibrillar structures
may be present (5). This type of tumor arises not only from
larger cartilage-bearing bronchi as an endobronchial polypoid
growth but also in the periphery of the lung forming a solid
mass, and is positively stained in many instances with
anti-lactoferrin immunohistochemically. It accounts for only
about 5% of adenocarcinoma cases.

3.4. Clara cell type

Peg-shaped cells with a tongue-like projection into the free
space from the level of junctional apparatus are arranged
either in a papillary fashion or bronchioloalveolar pattern.
Intranuclear inclusions positively stained with
anti-surfactant apoprotein are frequently noted. This type
probably arises from bronchioli and a solitary tumor mass
contains central fibrotic focus as a result of collapse of
alveoli previously occupied by the tumor cells. Sharp pleural
indentation is associated with central fibrosis. Electron
microscopically, tumor cells are rather rich in rough surfaced
endoplasmic reticulum and contain electron-dense secretory
granules of 200 to 900 nm in diameter, with or without
fingerprint-like structures (Fig. 4) (2, 3, 8, 9). Clara cell
type adenocarcinoma is the most common type adenocarcinoma,
accounting for more than 50% (some have reported up to 84%)
(2). No good marker substances are available at present.

3.5. Type II alveolar epithelial cell type

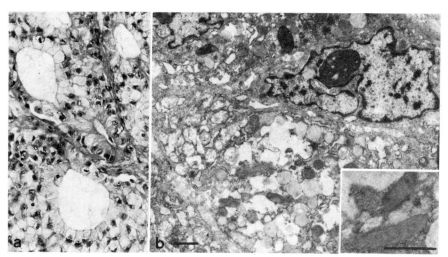

FIGURE 3. a) Histology of bronchial gland cell type discloses
mucus producing cells, which form tubular structures in areas.
b) Ultrastructurally, cytoplasm is filled with mucus granules
of varying density and occasional fibrillar structures
(inset).

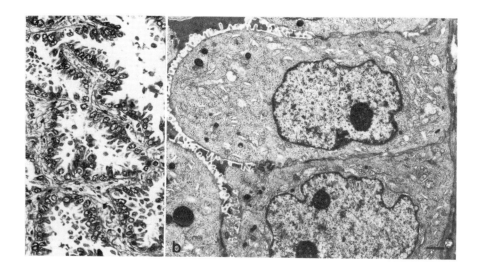

FIGURE 4. a) Histology of Clara cell type shows peg-shaped
cells, which are arranged in a papillary pattern. b)
Ultrastructurally cells are equipped with microvilli, rough
surface endoplasmic reticulum, and occasional electron dense
granules, which project from the level of junctional apparati
into the lumen.

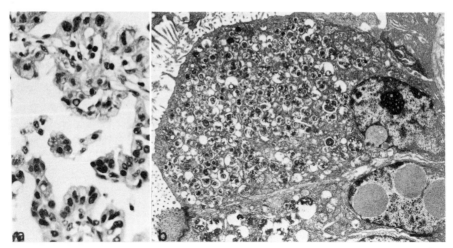

FIGURE 5. a) Histology of type II alveolar cell type reveals cuboidal cells with foamy cytoplasm arranged in a bronchioloalveolar pattern. b) Ultrastructurally cytoplasm is filled with lamellar bodies. Note amorphous nuclear inclusions.

   The histological structure of this cell type is identical to that of Clara cell type adenocarcinoma.   Diffuse lobar distribution of tumor cells may be seen.   Individual cells, however, are cuboidal with a dome-shaped free cell surface, and with some clear small vesicles in the cytoplasm, corresponding to which characteristic lamellar bodies are seen ultrastructurally (Fig. 5) (3, 10, 11).   This type of tumor is stained positively with anti-surfactant apoprotein (12).   In some tumors, type II alveolar-epithelial cell type tumor cells appear to co-exist with Clara cell type tumor cells (3).   Some of the tumors subtyped as Clara cell type by light and electron microscopy show a positive reaction with anti-surfactant apoprotein, the significance of which should be studied further.   Therefore, a distinct line between the Clara cell type and the type II alveolar cell type cannot be drawn.   The pure and well differentiated form of the latter type is infrequently seen.

3.6. Mixed cell type
   About 25% of adenocarcinomas less than 3 cm in diameter are of the mixed cell type.   Combinations of a & b, a & c, d & a or b, and d & e are noted.   The tumor cells that appear second or third in frequency are probably the result of metaplastic changes in the first cell type.
   Cytologic subclassification can be done in most well and moderately differentiated adenocarcinomas, but is difficult or impossible in some poorly differentiated forms.   The rate of agreement of subclassification by light and electron microscopy is very high, being over 90% in tumors of a single cell type (1).

4.MORPHOLOGIC FACTORS IN RELATION TO PROGNOSIS
   In adenocarcinomas less than 3 cm in diameter, postoperative
5-year survival rates were 68.4% in pathological Stage I
(n=57), 15.8% in Stage III (n=19) and 0% in Stage IV (n=4).
About one third of the cases of Stage Ia adenocarcinoma died
of the disease. Therefore, it is important to find
morphologic factors, other than T.N.M., which are related to
the prognosis of patients, in order to decide on postoperative
therapeutic procedures.
4.1.Histological and cytological subtypes
   In cases with a tumor less than 3 cm in diameter, the 5-year
survival rate of papillary adenocarcinoma was 50.7% (36/71)
and that of acinar type 41.7% (5/12). There was no case of
bronchioloalveolar carcinoma in this group. Cases with solid
carcinomas with mucus formation less than 3 cm in diameter
were also few in number, and 1 of 2 cases survived over 5
years.
   When analyzed according to cytological subtype the numbers
of cases of adenocarcinoma less than 3 cm in diameter are also
too small to assess with statistical significance. The 5-year
survival rate of cases of Clara cell type adenocarcinoma,
which were the largest in number was 54.3% (25/46), while that
of all adenocarcinoma was 49.4% (42/85).

4.2.Degrees of differentiation and cell atypia
   The highest 5-year survival rate in adenocarcinoma less than
3 cm in diameter was seen in well differentiated carcinoma
(64.1%), followed by moderately differentiated
(46.7%) and poorly differentiated (18.8%), and statistical
significance was only observed between the well differentiated
and the poorly differentiated groups (P<0.01) (Fig. 6). The

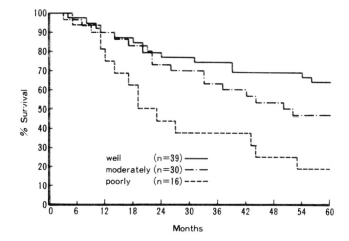

FIGURE 6. Survival curves in adenocarcinoma less than 3 cm in
diameter according to degree of histological differentiation.

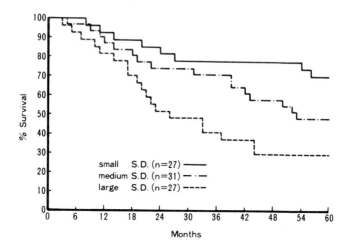

FIGURE 7. Survival curves in adenocarcinoma less than 3 cm in diameter according to the size of standard deviation of nuclear areas.

percentages in tumors less than 2 cm in diameter were 78.2% (n=37), 53.9% (n=27) and 28.3% (n=11), respectively (P<0.01).
    Similar results were obtained with the degree of cell atypia. The cell atypia was assessed by cytometric indices, that is, standard deviation of nuclear area and/or average nuclear area, which were graded respectively into 3 groups, small, medium and large nuclear areas and deviations. The smaller the index, the higher the 5-year survival rate. This inverse relationship had statistical significance. In terms of standard deviation the 5-year survival rates in adenocarcinoma less than 3 cm in diameter were 70.4% in a group with small deviation, 48.4% in a group with medium deviation and 29.6% in a group with large deviation. The difference between the two groups with small and large deviations was statistically significant (P<0.01) (Fig. 7). The 5-year survival for tumors less than 2 cm in diameter were 74.9% (n=26), 57.6% (n=25) and 52.3% (n=24), respectively (P< 0.05).

4.3.Vascular invasion
    The 5-year survival rate in tumors less than 2 cm in diameter was 83.8% in those without definite vascular invasion and 48.8% in those with evident vascular invasion. The difference was significant (P<0.01) (Fig. 8). In making this distinction, we did not specify the type of blood vessel, whether they were pulmonary arteries or veins, since it was sometimes difficult to identify vessels as such.

4.4.Mitotic index
    The 5-year survival rate of adenocarcinoma cases less than 3 cm was 75.0%, 50.0% and 22.2% in cases with mitotic indices of

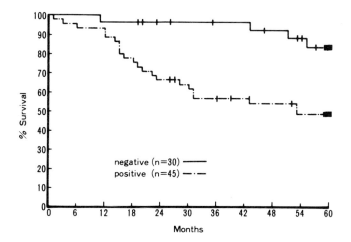

FIGURE 8. Survival curves in adenocarcinoma less than 2 cm in diameter, with and without vascular invasion.

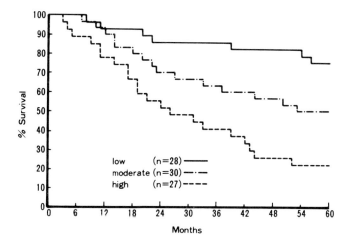

FIGURE 9. Survival curves in adenocarcinoma less than 3 cm in diameter, according to mitotic index.

below 0.5% (low), between 0.5 and 1.0% (moderate) and above 1.0% (high), respectively. The difference between the two groups with the low and high mitotic indices was significant (P<0.01) (Fig. 9) (1). The 5-year survival in cases with a tumor less than 2 cm in diameter and with a mitotic index of less than 0.35% was 81.7% (n=24), which was higher than those with an index of between 0.36 and 0.59% (n=26, 58.6%) and larger than 0.60% (n=25, 46.9%) (P<0.05).

28

A recently developed immunohistochemical method using
anti-bromodeoxyuridine (Budr) antibody can be applied to
surgical pathology either after preoperative intravenous
injection of Budr or incubation of tumor slices in Budr-
containing medium, which would enable us to easily identify
tumor cells synthesizing DNA (Fig. 10).

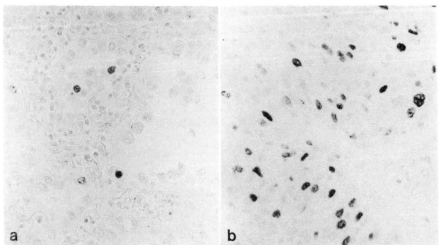

FIGURE 10. a) Budr-labelled nuclei are few in number in well
differentiated papillary adenocarcinoma, b) but many in poorly
differentiated adenocarcinoma (immunostain with anti-Budr).

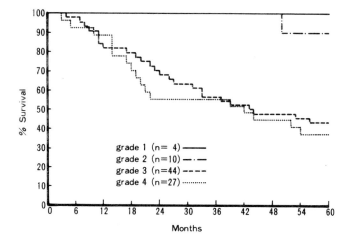

FIGURE 11. Survival curves in adenocarcinoma less than 3 cm in
diameter according to degree of stromal collagenization.

4.5.Degree of collagenization in stroma

Peripheral adenocarcinomas almost invariably contain central or subpleural anthracotic foci, where varying degrees of collagenization is noted.

The 5-year survival rate in cases of adenocarcinoma less than 3 cm in diameter with no fibrotic focus (grade 1) was 100% and that for cases with minimal collagenization in the stroma (grade 2) was 90%, which was higher than the rate for cases with definite collagenization with fibroblastic proliferation (grade 3) (43.2%) and hyalinization (grade 4) (37.0%) (P<0.01) (Fig. 11) (13).

In tumors less than 2 cm in diameter, the rates were 100% in grades 1 and 2 (n=5+8), 57.6% in grade 3 (n=47) and 46.7% in grade 4 (n=15). The difference was significant (P<0.01).

4.6.Host factors

Marked infiltration of T-zone histiocytes (Langerhans cells and their precursor, S100 protein and OKT 6 positive cells) (Fig. 12) in the primary tumor and in the regional lymph node (14) is associated with better prognosis. The 5-year survival rates were 70.8% with marked infiltration (more than 11 cells per high power field), 52.9% with moderate infiltration (2 to 10 cells) and 25.9% with no or slight infiltration (0-1 cell) in tumors of less than 3 cm, statistical difference being only observed between the marked and no or slight infiltration groups (P<0.01) (Fig. 13); and 71.9% (n=36) in a group with marked infiltration and 50.5% (n=36) in a group with no or slight infiltration in cases with tumors less than 2 cm in diameter. These differences were statistically significant

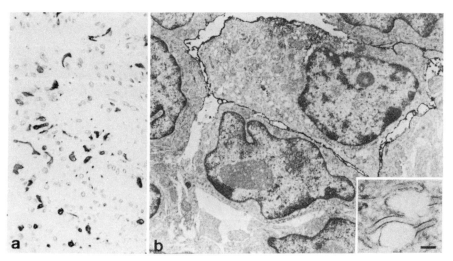

FIGURE 12. a) T-zone histiocytes in well differentiated adenocarcinoma (immunostain with OKT 6). b) Immuno-electron-microscopy with OKT 6 shows positive reaction in cell membrane of a cell in which the cytoplasm contains Birbeck granules (inset).

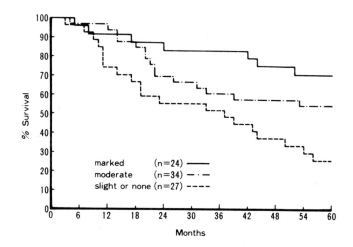

FIGURE 13. Survival curves in adenocarcinoma less than 3 cm in diameter according to degree of T-zone histiocyte infiltration in primary tumor.

TABLE 1.   Scoring of various prognostic factors

Factor	Score
Histological differentiation	
well	0
moderately	1
poorly	2
Nuclear atypia (standard deviation)	
small	0
medium	1
large	2
Mitotic index	
low	0
moderate	1
high	2
Scar grade	
Grade 1	0
Grade 2	1
Grade 3	2
Grade 4	3
Infiltration of T-zone histiocytes	
marked	0
moderate	1
slight or none	2

(P<0.05). The 5-year survival rate of cases with paracortical lymphocytic hyperplasia in the regional lymph node in Stage Ia adenocarcinoma (n=40) was significantly higher (75.0%) than in cases without hyperplasia (n=10, 40.0%) (P<0.05). However, such a correlation was not seen with regard to Stage Ib and II cases (n=22) or follicular hyperplasia (n=31:19) (1).

4.7. Scoring of morphologically identifiable prognostic factors
From the results shown herein, excluding the TNM factors, the morphological factors associated with better prognosis of patients, particularly in adenocarcinoma of less than 3 or 2 cm in diameter is well differentiated histology, lesser degree of nuclear atypia, fewer mitotic figures, no collagenization foci in stroma, frequent T-zone histiocytes in the primary tumor and paracortical lymph node hyperplasia in the regional lymph nodes. Scoring of these factors will contribute to the clinician's decision on the necessity and selection of post-operative adjuvant chemotherapy. Table 1 indicates an example of scoring of 5 morphological prognostic factors, and Fig. 14 reveals survival curves of 3 groups (Scores 0-4, 5-7 and 8-11) with tumors less than 3 cm in diameter (unpublished data). Although the survival curves were clearly separated, revealing the 5-year survival rates of 88.0, 48.7 and 4.8%, respectively, the validity of this approach should be confirmed by analyzing cases of adenocarcinoma in Stage I or Stage Ia. Accumulation of Stage Ia adenocarcinoma cases may also clarify the significance of histologic and cytologic subclassifications of adenocarcinoma.

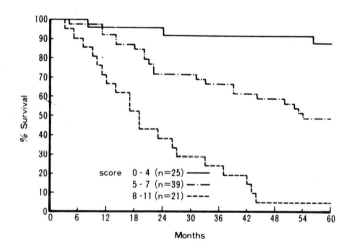

FIGURE 14. Survival curves in adenocarcinoma less than 3 cm in diameter according to score of five prognostic factors.

5. CONCLUSIONS

In this chapter, we presented a variety of morphologic factors related to the prognosis of patients with adenocarcinoma of the lung, apart from the presently widely used T.N.M factors. Materials used for the analysis were adenocarcinomas of less than 3 and 2 cm in diameter.

One of the factors we considered to be important was the cell type, the morphology of which was described briefly. However, the clinical significance of cytologic subtyping could not be proved because of the small number contained in many of the subgroups. In order to be used widely, identification of marker substances for each cell type, particularly for Clara cell type, is necessary. For this purpose, production of monoclonal antibodies against the differentiation antigens for each cell type is required.

Other factors, such as degrees of differentiation and cell atypia, vascular invasion, mitotic index, degree of collagenization in tumor stroma and host factors, were found to be of significance in predicting prognosis. The significance of some factors such as blood vessel invasion was reported by other investigators (15). Scoring of these factors may help the clinician's decision on the necessity and type of postoperative adjuvant chemotherapy, particularly in cases of Stage I or Stage Ia adenocarcinoma.

Although not stated in this chapter, as a result of efforts to detect small cancers located in the periphery of the lung, we have recently had occasion to observe lesions which were difficult to classify as either extremely well differentiated adenocarcinoma or as atypical adenomatous hyperplasia (or adenoma?). Although still few in number, there are cases in which adenocarcinoma appeared to have developed in such a lesion, simulating the adenoma-carcinoma sequence in the colo-rectum (16). The factor scores in those tumors were extremely low, so that a majority of those cases may be curable by lobectomy without mediastinal node dissection or even by partial lobectomy or segmentectomy in future.

REFERENCES

1. Shimosato Y: Lung cancer: Histogenesis, differentiation and prognostic factors. Tr Soc Pathol Jpn 72: 29-57, 1983. (in Japanese)
2. Kimula Y: A histochemical and ultrastructural study of adenocarcinoma of the lung. Am J Surg Pathol 2: 253-264, 1978.
3. Shimosato Y, Kodama T, Kameya T: Morphogenesis of peripheral type adenocarcinoma of the lung. In Shimosato Y, Melamed MR and Nettesheim P(eds): Morphogenesis of Lung Cancer, vol 1, 65-89. Boca Raton, Florida: CRC Press, Inc, 1982.
4. WHO: Histological Typing of Lung Tumours. 2nd edition, World Health Organization, Geneva, 1981.
5. Kodama T, Shimosato Y, Kameya T: Histology and ultrastructure of bronchogenic and bronchial gland adenocarcinomas (including adenoid cystic and mucoepidermoid carcinomas) in relation to histogenesis. In

Shimosato Y, Melamed MR and Nettesheim P(eds):
Morphogenesis of Lung Cancer, vol 1, 147-166, Boca Raton,
Florida: CRC Press, Inc, 1982.

6. Kodama T, Shimosato Y, Koide T, et al: Endobronchial
polypoid adenocarcinoma of the lung. Histological and
ultrastructural studies of five cases. Am J Surg Pathol 8:
845-854, 1984.

7. Bedrossian CWM, Weilbacher DG, Bentinck DC, Greenberg SD:
Ultrastructure of human bronchioloalveolar cell carcinoma.
Cancer 36: 1399-1413, 1975.

8. Montes M, Binette JP, Adler RH, Guarino R: Clara cell
adenocarcinoma, light and electron microscopic studies. Am
J Surg Pathol 1: 245-253, 1977.

9. Jacques J, Currie W: Bronchiolo-alveolar carcinoma. A
Clara cell tumor. Cancer 40: 2171-2180, 1977.

10. Torikata C, Ishiwata K: Intranuclear tubular structures
observed in the cells of an alveolar cell carcinoma of the
lung. Cancer 40: 1194-2101, 1977.

11. Morningstar WA, Hassan MO: Bronchioloalveolar carcinoma
with nodal metastases. An ultrastructural study. Am J Surg
Pathol 3: 273-278, 1979.

12. Singh G, Katyal SL, Torikata C: Carcinoma of type II
pneumocytes. Immunodiagnosis of a subtype of
bronchiolo-alveolar carcinomas. Am J Pathol 102: 195-208,
1981.

13. Shimosato Y, Hashimoto T, Kodama T, et al: Prognostic
implications of fibrotic focus (scar) in small peripheral
lung cancers. Am J Surg Pathol 4: 365-373, 1980.

14. Watanabe S, Sato Y, Kodama T, Shimosato Y:
Immunohistochemical study with monoclonal antibodies on
immune response in lung cancers. Cancer Res 43: 5883-5889,
1983.

15. Spjut HJ, Roper CL, Butcher HRJr: Pulmonary cancer and its
prognosis. A study of the relationship of certain factors
to survival of patients treated by pulmonary resection.
Cancer 14: 1251-1258, 1961.

16. Shimosato Y, Kodama T: Low grade malignant and benign
tumor. In McDowell E(ed): Lung Carcinomas, Edingburgh:
Churchill Livingstone, in press.

PATHOLOGY OF   SMALL CELL CARCINOMA OF THE LUNG-CHANGING CONCEPTS

M.J.MATTHEWS

1. INTRODUCTION

In the past decade, impressive gains have been made in the
diagnosis,   staging and treatment of small cell lung cancer (SCCL).
Much of this improvement has been possible due to the World Health
Organization's (WHO) Lung Cancer Classification (1) and the establishment of light microscopic criteria for the various types and
subtypes of lung cancer.   Such criteria became particularly important when it was appreciated that SCLC tumors, in contrast to
non-small cell lung cancers (N-SCLC), had an impressive objective
response to chemotherapy and/or radiotherapy protocols (2).

With acceptance of morphologic criteria by a broad segment of
the pathology community,   an   impressive   degree   of   consistency,
reliability and reproducibility in the light microscopic diagnosis
of SCLC has become possible.   It is reported that appropriate tissue
diagnoses can be made consistently in cooperative oncology groups
in up to 94% of cases (3,4).   The accuracy of diagnosing cytologic
material by cell type approaches 99% in some reports (5,6).   With
such results,   comparability   of   treatment   and   survival   data   of
patients becomes realistic.   In spite of this degree of accuracy
or consistency in the diagnosis of SCLC, little agreement has been
achieved in the interpretation of its various subtypes.

Electron microscopic and immunohistochemical technics have been
utilized to identify ultrastructural and biochemical properties of
SCLC (7-9).   Biochemical and biologic studies of tissue cell cultures and nude mice heterotransplants have confirmed the amine con-
tent/ amine precursor uptake and decarboxylation (APUD) potential
and nature of SCLC tumors (10, 11) These studies have also, con-
vincingly, confirmed the morphogenesis of lung cancers, i.e., a
progenitor cell of entodermal origin probably gives rise to all
lung carcinomas regardless of cell type.

Such information requires changes in concepts in both the
clinical and pathology communities.   An impressive amount of data
has accumulated which suggests that biochemical and biologic data
heretofore considered pathognomonic for SCLC tumors are applicable
to atypical carcinoids and some N-SCLC tumors.   The oncology
community must be aware of these variants and develop protocols
designed to diagnose and treat them.   The pathology community
must recognize these variants, as well, and distinguish

them from the classic SCCL. There is growing recognition that there is no difference in behavior of the classic SCCL subtypes (12-14).

This report will summarize historical concepts of the morphology of SCCL. A short description of light microscopic criteria for tissue and cytologic diagnoses of SCLC and its variants will be given. Pathologic and clinical factors which influence response to therapy and survival will be discussed. The current role and value of electron microscopy, immunohistochemistry and experimental pathology in the diagnosis of this tumor will be addressed. An attempt will be made to define the interrelationships of lung tumors.

2. MORPHOLOGY OF SCCL

2.1 HISTORICAL CONCEPTS:

Barnard (15) identified SCLC as a carcinoma rather than a mediastinal sarcoma because of small foci of squamous nests, tubules or giant cells identified in these tumors, features which suggested their epithelial nature. In 1967, the WHO Lung Cancer Classification was published under the direction of Dr. L. Kreyberg (1). Four subtypes of SCLC were defined, based on nuclear size and contours (lymphocytelike, polygonal, fusiform and "others"). In 1972, the pathology panel of the Working Party for Therapy of Lung Cancer (WP-L) collated these groups into lymphocytelike and intermediate subtypes (16). In 1977, a reconvened panel of pathologists recommended that SCLC be divided into 3 subtypes oat-cell/lymphocyte-like ; intermediate and combined (SCLC tumors combined with frank adenocarcinoma or squamous cell carcinoma)(17). It was also recommended that small cell tumors with large cell component be considered a subset of the intermediate group, to assure its appropriate treatment.

2.2 MORPHOLOGIC CRITERIA:

2.21 Tissue Diagnoses:

Approximately 93-95% of SCLC are of a classic type, regardless of whether the tumor is interpreted as lymphocyte-like (oat cell) or intermediate. Small cell carcinomas, regardless of subtype, are identified by their nuclear characteristics. Cells measure 12-20 microns, tend to be arranged in clusters, have oval to spindled to rounded nuclei, with chromatin granules distributed in a fine or course pattern throughout the nucleus. Nucleoli are small and indistinct. Rare prominent nucleoli may be observed per low-power field. Numerous mitoses are present. Cytoplasm is usually scanty, resulting in molding of adjoining cells. Neoplastic cells are arranged in variable patterns, in nests, cords, trabeculae or sheets, separated by a thin fibrovascular stroma. Host response (plasma cells, lymphocytes or desmoplasia) is usually minimal or absent.

In areas of massive necrosis, DNA material may be seen deposited on elastic fibrils of ghosts of preexisting blood vessels. In fiberoptic bronchial biopsies, neoplastic cells are small, rounded, hyperchromatic and frequently show crushing effect secondary to instrumentation. Cells measure at least twice the size of identifiable lymphocytes. Mitoses are difficult to identify. Occasional tubules, squamous nests or giant cells may be identified in surgical specimens, such as lymph node or lung biopsies.

A small percentage of SCLC by light microscopy, estimated to be 6%, contain significant clusters of cells with abundant cytoplasm and prominent nucleoli. Such tumors have been defined as mixed small cell/large cell tumors (18). A much smaller percentage of tumors, estimated to be less than 1%, have frank squamous or adenocarcinomatous elements, in addition to small cell neoplasm. These latter tumors are most frequently identified , premortem, in surgical lung resections.

2.22 Cytologic Diagnoses

Cytologic diagnoses of SCLC is based on criteria similar to tissue diagnoses. In postbronchoscopy sputa and bronchial washings, neoplastic cells are twice the size of a lymphocyte, have dense hyperchromatic nuclei, are clustered and show nuclear molding. Identification of distinct neoplastic nuclear characteristics is not otherwise possible in many of these specimens. To the contrary, in aspirates of metastatic subcutaneous or superficial lymph node masses and bronchial brushings, cytologic diagnoses are facilitated by the well preserved nuclear chromatin pattern, cellular clustering and molding and absence of prominent nucleoli.

2.23 Problems in Diagnosis

A number of caveats must be given in the tissue and cytologic interpretation of SCLC.

1. Problems which can be resolved readily in the light microscopic diagnosis of classic SCLC relate, for the most part, to inadequacy of sampling of tumor, improper handling, fixation and staining of tissue or cytologic material and inconsistent application of light microscopic criteria.

Problems which loom in the future relate to identification of the mixed small-cell/large cell tumors; the distinction of some SCLC tumors from atypical carcinoids and the increasing evidence that some N-SCLC tumors, in fact, have APUD (biochemical/biologic neuroendocrine) features. The treatment of choice and evaluation of response to therapy and survival of these variant groups will require protocols by multiple cooperative groups who have the expertise to diagnose and treat these patients.

2. It is impossible to distinguish neoplastic nuclear characteristics in some cytologic specimens, beyond recognizing their nuclear hyperchromasia, molding and clustering. The "ink-dot" hyperchromasia and clustering of neoplastic cells in sputa, in particular, are considered diagnostic of small cell malignancies. It is worthwhile remarking, however, that these cells are hypoxic and degenerated.

3. Interpretation of transthoracic needle biopsies permits a diagnosis of malignancy. However, not infrequently, material is inadequate to distinguish cell type. Often the material obtained by these procedures represents a necrotic central focus of tumor. Neoplastic cells, in such circumstances, have dense hyperchromatic nuclei and indistinct cytoplasm. Cellular clustering permits a diagnosis of an epithelial malignancy. Because of the hyperchromasia and scanty cytoplasm, such tumors may be interpreted as SCLC. Cytologic diagnoses should not be accepted in such instances for protocol purposes unless confirmed by tissue diagnosis.

4. In a small percentage of cases, neoplasms quite characteristic of SCLC on Papanicolau stains may be interpreted as large cell lung cancer on Giemsa/Wright stains. It is important that this anomaly be recognized and that tissue diagnosis be obtained before a patient is placed on protocol.

5. There is a growing awareness that a number of N-SCLC tumors have endocrine trabecular patterns by light microscopy and neuroendocrine features identified by special silver stains, by immunohistochemistry and/or other biological and biochemical technics. It is difficult, at present, to estimate the percentage of these tumors in the total lung cancer population. The cytologic diagnoses of some of these tumors are fraught with problems. Neoplastic cells, particularly in pleural fluid, tend to be small and clustered, have no distinct neoplastic characteristics and may be indistinguishable from mesothelial clusters. Prominent nucleoli are not identifiable in the papillary clusters. In one such recent case, a patient presented with a peripheral subpleural nodule, massive pleural effusion, multiple lytic bony lesions and skin and subcutaneous nodules. Pleural fluid was interpreted as adenocarcinoma on the basis of small tight papillary clusters. Biopsy of several skin lesions were interpreted as adenocarcinoma. Mucicarmine and Pascual stains of pleural fluid cell blocks were minimally positive. To the contrary, skin and subcutaneous metastases were exuberantly positive for granules on Pascual silver and chromogranin stains.

6. In the past four years, an increasing number of atypical small cell tumors, carcinoid-like tumors as well as N-SCCL tumors with neuroendocrine features have been reviewed in the NCI-Navy MOB. Initially, it was thought that these "odd-balls" were coming to us because there are many oncologists in the medical community to care for the

patient with classic small cell cancer. Much of the increase, on the contrary, reflects the efforts of the MOB's experimental research division which performs many biologic, biochemical and immunohistochemical studies on SCLC as well as N-SCLC tumors. It is possible that within the next decade or two, these studies will lead to an entirely different approach to the diagnosis and treatment of all lung cancers.

3. MORPHOLOGIC FACTORS INFLUENCING PATIENT RESPONSE RATE AND SURVIVAL

In an 8 year period, 360 patients with SCLC were evaluated for staging and treatment purposes at the NCI-VA Medical Oncology Branch (13). Of 103 patients diagnosed as having classic small cell carcinoma, either lymphocyte or intermediate type, there was no difference in patient characteristics, extent of disease, metastatic behavior, response to high dose chemotherapy or median survival. Median survival was over 10 months for both cell subtypes and objective response rate for each subtype was 90%. Patients with a 0-1 performance status, with limited disease had a median survival of over 17 months. Of 252 patients treated on various chemotherapy/radiotherapy protocols, 14 (5.6%) are alive and well over 5 years (median 7.4 with a range of 6.4 to 11.3 years). These patients may be considered cured of their disease (19).

To the contrary, 18 patients identified prospectively as having mixed SC/LC tumors were treated on similar chemotherapy protocols (18). There was no significant difference in patient characteristics, extent of disease or metastatic behavior. On the other hand, the objective response rate of these tumors was 56%; the median survival 6 months, and a particularly poor survival was identified in patients who presented with good performance status and limited disease (7 months as compared to 17.5 months). To the contrary, 2 of these patients survived over one year and one of the patients is still alive over 5 years.

An insufficient number of patients with atypical carcinoid/small cell or N-SCLC APUD tumors have been studied or treated to date to comment on natural behavior or response to therapy of this subset of tumors.

4. ROLE OF IMMUNOHISTOCHEMISTRY, ELECTRON MICROSCOPY AND CELL BIOLOGY IN THE DIAGNOSIS OF SCLC.

4.1 GENERAL COMMENTS:

There is little doubt that cell biology, immunohistochemistry and electron microscopy have provided much insight into the biochemical nature of SCLC as well as the histogenesis and precise ultrastructural characteristics of all lung cancers. The latter two technics, when positive, can be also immensely helpful in diagnosing tumors which defy light microscopic interpretation. At present, however, the state of art leaves much to be desired. Questions must be raised regarding economic feasibility; whether these technics can assure consistency and reliability of interpretation between institutions and countries; whether the multiplicity of classifications based on these technics have any clinical relevance; and whether these technics can be more predictive of response to therapy and improved survival than their light microscopic counterparts in the diagnosis of SCLC patients.

4.2 IMMUNOHISTOCHEMISTRY:

Sappino et al identified 9/45 cases of SCLC which contained keratin immunoreactive cells in at least a small portion of the tumors (20). Two-thirds of patients who had keratin markers and one-third of patients whose tumors lacked keratin reactivity had complete responses to chemotherapy. The authors felt that the presence or absence of this reactivity did not appear to influence or correlate with extent of disease at presentation, response to therapy or survival of small cell patients. Gould et al. have used a battery of specific antibodies (ACTH, bombesin, calcitonin, leu-enkephalin, gastrin, glucagon, somatotostatin, serotonin and VIP) to identify secretory granules in neuroendocrine tumors (9). Carcinoid tumors showed the most reactivity (2-5 hormones were identified per tumor, particularly bombesin, serotonin, calcitonin, leu enkephalin, somatostatin and VIP). To the contrary, classic small cell tumors were minimally positive, faint and sporadic (probably related to the fact that materials were bronchial biopsies and fixed in formalin rather than in Bouin's solution). Kameya et al (21) reported similar immunohistochemistry results. In spite of appropriate fixation, only 2/16 cases of SCLC showed positive imm oreactivity, although 5/6 specimens submitted for radioimmunoassay were positive.

4.3 ELECTRON MICROSCOPY:

Multiple reports document the presence of glandular (microvilli) or squamous elements at ultrastructural levels, with or without associated dense core granules in tumors diagnosed as classic SCLC by light microscopy (7,22,23). McDowell and Trump (24) have reported elements representing the three cell types in a single cell. Similar tripartite elements have been recently identified in a small cell culture line (10). Mackay (7) estimates that the majority of small cell tumors contain dense core (neurosecretory) granules. This is particularly true if adequate diagnostic material is received and appropriately fixed. Sidhu (23), working retrospectively with formalin fixed materials and bronchial biopsies, identified dense core granules in only 30% of cases diagnosed by light microscopy as SCLC. Kameya et al (21) were able to identify dense core granules in only 40% of similar biopsy materials studied by EM. Li et al (25) reported that 2/3 of patients with a light microscopic diagnosis of SCLC had dense core granules by EM. Survival appeared to be related more to the stage of disease than presence of dense core granules. The authors infer that if dense core granules are not identified by EM, the light microscopic interpretation is incorrect.

It would appear that adequate sampling and proper fixation are as critical for immunohistochemistry and electron microscopy as they are for light microscopic interpretation. These technics, at present, are not economically feasible as routine procedures. Much work must be done prospectively to improve the quality and accessibility of antibodies used in immunohistochemistry as well as the quality of materials submitted for EM. It would appear, at present, that consistency and reliability in the diagnosis of SCLC does not yet approach that of light microscopic interpretation.

4.4 EXPERIMENTAL PATHOLOGY

At the NCI-Navy Medical Oncology Branch   , continuous cell line cultures and nude mice xenografts have been established from the tumors of 50 patients diagnosed as SCLC by light microscopy (26). These lines have been analyzed for their light and electron microscopic characteristics, nude mice tumorigenicity, and hormone and enzyme production. Of the 50 tumors, 35 (70%) have shown classic morphology, and produce high levels of dopa decarboxylase, bombesin, neuron specific enolase and the BB isoenzyme of creatine kinase (CK-BB). Fifteen of the cell lines have been considered either biochemical or morphologic variants. Both variants have altered biochemical profiles, in that essentially no dopa decarboxylase or bombesin can be identified and dense core granules are markedly reduced or absent in the cell lines. On the other hand, the tumors have high levels of neuron specific enolase and CK-BB, show the cytogenetic anomaly of small cell tumors (P3 deletion) and are frequently associated with greatly amplified levels of the c myc oncogene. Cell lines considered biochemical variants retain characteristic SCLC morphology and growth characteristics. Cell lines considered morphologic variants, to the contrary, have or develop features of large cell carcinoma (large cells with abundant cytoplasm and prominent nucleoli), have altered growth patterns, clone readily and have more rapid doubling times. Ultrastructures of these latter tumors contain squamous and/or glandular elements.

5. INTERRELATIONSHIP OF SCLC AND OTHER LUNG CANCERS

From the earliest recognition of SCLC, squamous or glandular elements or anaplastic large cells have been identified and appreciated. appreciated. Although it is estimated that 6% of small cell tumors have a significant large cell component at diagnosis, at autopsy N-SCLC components can be identified in over 1/3 of treated cases (27).

The recognition that classic SCLC tumors may have ultrastructural characteristics of all 4 lung cancer cell types would seem to support the consideration that all lung tumors are derived from a common precursor/progenitor cell. The in-vitro morphologic variants described above appear to replicate, in a sense, the clinical and pathologic behavior of patients with mixed small cell large cell tumors. The morphologic transformation and loss of APUD properties by SCCL suggest the loss of differentiation and function of a highly complex cell. It is possible to speculate that over time, or in response to therapy, that sensitive neoplastic small cells are depleted and that the progenitor cells are stimulated to differentiate in other pathways.

The large cell tumors discussed above are indistinguishable from the large cell components present in all poorly differentiated carcinomas. It would seem almost inevitable that the progenitor neoplastic cells have been programmed to mature and function as reserve, columnar goblet, squamous or neuroendocrine type cells. The entodermal origin of all these tumors is therefore presumed. Such an interpretation permits a better understanding of the interrelationship of all lung cancers and the mixed histologies, in particular.

In response to some of the problems cited above, and to clarify interpretation of the classic SCLC, a pathology panel (12) of the IASLC which met in Gleneagles, Scotland, in September, 1984, recommended the following:

1. The term SCLC should replace the terms "oat-cell, lymphocyte-like and intermediate" for all tumors which have no significant (less than 1%) N-SCLC elements.

2. Two variants of SCLC should be recognized.

    a. Mixed small cell/large cell.
    b. Combined small cell carcinomas.

The recommendations were made in an attempt to remove from dispute the classic SCLC subtypes and to focus on the small percentage of variant tumors which create problems by light microscopy.

REFERENCES:

1. Kreyberg, L.: Histological Typing of Lung Tumors. International
   Histologic Classification of Tumors, Geneva. World Health Organization, 1967.

2. Minna, J.D., Higgins, G.A. and Glatstein, E.J.: Cancer of the lung,
   in Principles and Practice of Oncology, (V.T. DeVita, S. Hellman and
S. Rosenberg, eds.) Philadelphia, J.P. Lippincott, 1982, 396-473.

3. Janis, M., Matthews, M.D., Bonfiglio, T., et al: Consistency in the
   diagnosis of small cell lung cancer. Proc. II World Conference on
Lung Cancer, Copenhagen, 1980, 179.

4. Vollmer, R.T., Ogden, L., Crissman, J.D.: Separation of small cell
   from non-small cell lung cancer. The Southeastern Cancer Study Group
pathologists' experience. Arch. Pathol. Lab. Med. 108 (10):792-794, 1984.

5. Mitchell, M.L., King, D.E., Bonfiglio, T.A., et al: Pulmonary fine
   needle aspiration cytopathology--a five year correlation study. Acta
Cytol. 28(1): 72-76, 1984.

6. Ng, A.B. and Horak, G.C.: Factors significant in diagnostic accuracy
   of lung cytology in bronchial washings and sputum specimens. Acta
Cytol. 27: 391-396, 1983.

7. Mackay, B. Ultrastructure of lung neoplasms, in Lung Cancer, Clinical
   Diagnosis and Treatment, (M.J.Straus, ed.) 2nd edition, New York,
Grune and Stratton, 1983, 85-96.

8. Gould, V.E. and Chejfec, T.: Ultrastructural and biochemical analysis
of undifferentiated pulmonary carcinomas. Human Pathol 9:377-384, 1978.

9. Gould, V.E., Linnoila, I., Warren, H., et al: Neuroendocrine cells
   and neuroendocrine neoplasms of the lung. Pathol. Annual 18 (11):
287-330, 1983.

10. Gazdar, A.F.: The biology of endocrine tumors of the lung, in The
    Endocrine Lung in Health and Disease, Philadelphia, W.B. Saunders,
1984, 448-457.

11. Carney, D.N., Gazdar, A.F., Bepler, G., et al: Establishment and
identification of small cell lung cancer cell lines having classic and
varfiant features. Cancer Research. In press.

12. Yesner, R.: Classification of lung cancer histology. New England
    J. Med. 312 (10): 652-653, 1985.

13. Carney, D.N., Matthews, M.J., Ihde, D.C., et al: Influence of histologic subtype of small cell carcinoma of the lung on clinical presentation, response to therapy and survival. J. National Cancer Institute, 65: 1225-1229, 1980.

14. Vollmer, R.T., Birch, R., Ogden, L., et al: Subclassification of small cell cancer of the lung. The Southeastern Cancer Study Group experience. Human Pathol. 16(3): 247-252, 1985.

15. Barnard, W.G.: The nature of the "oat-celled" sarcoma of the mediastinum. J. Pathol. Bact. 29: 241-244, 1926.

16. Matthews, M.J.: Morphologic classification of bronchogenic carcinoma. Cancer Chemother. Rep. 4(3): 63-67, 1973.

17. Yesner, R. and Sobin, L.: Histologic Typing of Lung Tumors, 2nd edition; International Histologic Classification of Tumors. Geneva, World Health Organization, 1981.

18. Radice, P.A., Matthews, M.J., Ihde, D.C., et al: The clinical behavior of "mixed" small cell/large cell bronchogenic carcinoma compared to "pure" small cell subtype. Cancer 50: 2894-2902, 1982.

19. Johnson, B.E., Ihde, D.C., Bunn, P.A., et al: Five to eleven year follow-up of small cell lung cancer patients treated with combination chemotherapy with or without irradiation. Potential cures, chronic toxicities and late relapses. American J. Med. In press.

20. Sappino, A.P., Ellison, M.K.L., and Gusterson, B.A.: Immunohisto-chemical localization of keratin in small cell carcinoma of the lung. Correlation with response to combination chemotherapy. European J. Cancer Clin. Oncol. 19(10): 1365-1370, 1983.

21. Kameya, T., Kodama, T., and Shimosato, Y.: Ultrastructure of small cell carcinoma of the lung (oat and intermediate types) in relation to histogenesis and carcinoid tumors, in Morphogenesis of Lung Cancer, Volume II (Y. Shimosato, M.R. Melamed and F. Nettesheim eds.) Boca Raton, CRC Press, 1982, 15-44.

22. Churg, A., Johnston, W.H. and Stulbarg, M.: Small cell, squamous and mixed small cell squamous-small cell anaplastic carcinomas of the lung. Am. J. Surg. Pathol. 4: 255-263, 1980.

23. Sidhu, G.S.: The ultrastructure of malignant epithelial neoplasms. Pathol. Annual 17: 235-266, 1982.

24. McDowell, E.M. and Trump, B.F.: Pulmonary small cell carcinoma showing tripartite differentiation in individual cells. Human Pathol. 12: 286-294, 1981.

25. Li, W., Hammer, S.P., Jolly, P.C., et al: Unpredictable course of small cell undifferentiated lung cancer. J. Thorac. Cardiovasc. Surg. 81: 34-43, 1981.

26. Gazdar, A.F., Carney, D.N., Nau, M.M., et al: Characterization of variant subclasses of cell lines derived from small cell lung cancer, having distinctive biochemical, morphologic and growth properties. Cancer Res. In press.

27. Matthews, M.J.: Effects of therapy on the morphology and behavior of small cell carcinoma of the lung: A clinicopathologic study, in Lung Cancer, Progress in Therapeutic Research, (F. Muggia and M. Rozencweig, eds.) New York, Raven Press, 1979, 155-164.

SMALL CELL CARCINOMAS VERSUS (ATYPICAL) CARCINOIDS

B.CORRIN

1.SMALL CELL CARCINOMAS AND TYPICAL CARCINOIDS
    Because small cell carcinomas sometimes show histological features sug-
gestive of carcinoid differentiation and because these two tumours show a
similar spectrum of ectopic endocrine syndromes,Bensch et al (1) examined
a series of lung carcinomas by electron microscopy, systematically searching
for ultrastructural features of carcinoid tumours. It was already known
that bronchial carcinoids were characterized by numerous small (150-250 nm
diameter) dense core neurosecretory granules. Such granules were found in
small numbers in a few cells of all small cell carcinomas examined but not
in any undifferentiated large cell lung carcinomas. Mattori et al (2) inde-
pendently reported similar results. Cells with similar neurosecretory granules were identified in bronchial glands (3) and subsequently in the surface epithelium of the airways (4) and it was proposed that carcinoid tumours
and small cell carcinomas were the locally invasive and highly malignant
varieties respectively of tumours derived from these "Kultschitsky-type"
cells (1). Subsequently a small proportion of small cell carcinomas have
been shown to possess squamous or glandular features on electron microscopy (5-8) and dense core granules have been identified in a few large cell
carcinomas, adenocarcinomas and epidermoid carcinomas (9-11), whilst even
tripartite differentiation, involving squamous, mucous and neuroendocrine
features, has been identified in individual tumour cells (11). These excep-
tions are however all relatively rare and the close histogenetic relationship between carcinoid tumours and the majority of small cell carcinomas,
established nearly twenty years ago, has not been seriously challenged.
Evidence for the relationship from recent immunocytochemical studies is
conflicting however. Sheppard et al (12) found neurone-specific enolase,
a marker isoenzyme of neuro-endocrine cells throughout the body, in 16 of
18 pulmonary carcinoids and in 17 of 31 small cell carcinomas but in no
other variety of lung tumour. Others however report that this enzyme is
present in many non neuroendocrine tumours (13-15).

1.1. Etiology
    Although small cell carcinoma and carcinoids are closely related histo-
genetically, there are profound differences between these two tumours. The
well known association of cigarette smoking with small cell carcinoma is
not a feature of pulmonary carcinoids. In line with this, carcinoids lack
the male preponderance shown by small cell carcinomas, and occur about a
decade earlier: the male/female ratio is 0.8 and the peak age of onset 51
years (16).

1.2. Behaviour
    In behaviour too, these two tumours are dramatically different. The high-
ly aggressive growth pattern of small cell carcinoma (2%, 5-year survival)
(17) contrasts with the relatively benign behaviour of carcinoids. Although
the latter are no longer regarded as adenomas, the growth of typical carcinoids is slow and their propensity to metastasise low. In a review of
190 cases of bronchopulmonary carcinoid, Godwin found that in 79 per cent
the tumour was confined to the lung and there was a 96 per cent 5-year
survival, 15 per cent showed regional lymph node involvement and had a

71 per cent 5-year survival,and 5 per cent had distant metastases and an 11 per cent 5-year survival (16).

2. ATYPICAL CARCINOIDS

2.1. Behaviour
The relatively rare atypical variety of pulmonary carcinoid has a worse prognosis than the typical carcinoid tumour. In one study of atypical carcinoid tumours, regional or distant metastases developed in 70 per cent of patients and 30 per cent died of their tumour (18), whilst in another 8 of 17 patients died of their tumour, the mean survival being 10 months (19). Atypical carcinoids are therefore intermediate in their behaviour between the usual pulmonary carcinoid and small cell carcinoma (Table 1).

TABLE 1

	Carcinoid Typical	Carcinoid Atypical	Small Cell Carcinoma
Behaviour			
Local invasion	Present	Present	Present
Lymphatic metastases	Occasional	Frequent	Normal
Distant metastases	Rare	45-70%	95-100%

Gould et al advocate a new nomenclature which acknowledges the close relationship of atypical carcinoid and small cell carcinoma: in their classification, small cell carcinomas are named neuroendocrine carcinomas of small cell type, and atypical carcinoids are termed well differentiated neuroendocrine carcinomas (20). Because of their intermediate growth pattern, behaviour and prognosis, atypical carcinoids must be recognised by the histopathologist and distinguished from both typical carcinoids and small cell carcinomas.

2.2. Histological appearances
Typical carcinoids consist of small regular cells with vesicular nuclei and eosinophilic granular cytoplasm. The cells are usually arranged in a moisaic or trabecular pattern, or less commonly an adeno-papillary arrangement with mucus secretion (21, 22). Mixtures of these patterns are common. Cytological variants include the uncommon clear cell carcinoids (23),large eosinophilic cell or oncocytoid carcinoids (24-25) and spindle cell carcinoids (27,28), this last pattern being found particularly in peripheral tumours. In all these varieties of carcinoid, there is no necrosis and mitotic figures are generally not observed.
Atypical carcinoids show the trabecular or mosaic arrangement, and well demarcated edge, of typical carcinoids, but also display cellular pleomorphism, nuclear irregularity, mitotic activity and necrosis (18, 19, 27). Focal loss of histological pattern is a further feature of atypical carcinoids (Table 2).

TABLE 2.

	Carcinoid Typical	Carcinoid Atypical	Small Cell Carcinoma
Histology			
Architecture	Well organised	Focal loss	None
Necrosis	None	Focal	Abundant
DNA on vessels	None	None	Present
Cytology			
Mitoses	Not seen	Common	Numerous
Pleomorphism	Absent	Moderate	Marked
Argyrophilia	Common	Variable	Rare

2.3. Etiology

Sixteen of the 17 atypical carcinoids described by Mills (19) developed in cigarette smokers yet, as with behaviour and histological structures, atypical carcinoids are intermediate in sex incidence and age distribution (2 to 1 male predominance, mean age 58 years) between typical carcinoids (slight female predominance, mean age 51 years) and small cell carcinomas (marked, but diminishing male preponderance, mean age 61 years) (Table 3).

TABLE 3.

	Carcinoid Typical	Carcinoid Atypical	Small Cell Carcinoma
Etiology			
Role of smoking	None	Strong	Strong
Male/female ratio	0.8 : 1	2 : 1	4 : 1
Mean age (yrs)	51	58	61

2.4. Ultrastructure

Another intermediate feature is the number of neurosecretory granules evident by electron microscopy. They are less numerous in atypical than typical carcinoids, but more easily found than in small cell carcinomas. The size of the granules varies but in atypical carcinoids they approximate more to the smaller 80-140 nm granules of small cell carcinomas than the 150-250 nm granules of typical carcinoids (20) (Table 4).

TABLE 4.

	Carcinoid Typical	Carcinoid Atypical	Small Cell Carcinoma
Ultrastructure			
Granule numbers	Many	Moderate	Scanty
Granule size (nm)	150-250	80-140	80-140

3. CONCLUSION

Pathologically, typical carcinoids, atypical carcinoids and small cell carcinomas comprise a spectrum of neuroendocrine neoplasms(26) but for practical purposes the histopathologist has to place individual tumours in a particular category. Necrosis, abundant mitoses, focal loss of architecture and cellular pleomorphism help to distinguish atypical carcinoids from small cell carcinomas.

REFERENCES

1. Bensch KG, Corrin B, Pariente R, Spencer H: Oat cell carcinoma of the lung. Its origin and relationship to bronchial carcinoid. Cancer 22: 1163-1172,1968.
2. Hattori S, Matsuda M, Tatieshi R, Tatsumi N, Terazawa T: Oat-cell carcinoma of the lung containing serotonin granules. Gann 59:123-129, 1968.
3. Bensch KG, Gordon GB, Miller LR: Electron microscopic and biochemica studies on the bronchial carcinoid tumour. Cancer 18:592-602,1965.
4. Gmelic JT, Bensch KG, Liebow AA: Cells of Kultschitzky type in bronchioles and their relation to the origin of peripheral carcinoid tumour. Laboratory Investigation 17:88-98,1967.
5. Churg A, Johnston WH, Stulbarg M: Small cell squamous and mixed small cell squamous - small cell anaplastic carcinomas of the lung. American Journal of Surgical Pathology 4:255-263,1980.
6. Leong SYL, Canny AR: Small cell anaplastic carcinoma of the lung with glandular and squamous differentiation. American Journal of Surgical Pathology 5:307-309,1981.
7. Saba SR, Azar HA, Richman AV, Solomon DA, Spurlock RG, Mardelli IG, Kasnic C: Dual differentiation in small cell carcinoma (oat cell carcinoma) of the lung. Ultrastructural Pathology 2:131-138,1981.
8. Bolen JW, Thorning D: Histo genetic classification of lung carcinomas. Small cell carcinomas studied by light and electron microscopy. Journal Submicroscopy & Cytology 14:499-514,1982.
9. McDowell EM, Trump BF: Pulmonary small cell carcinoma showing tripartite differentiation in individual cells. Human Pathology 12: 286-294,1981.
10. Saba SR, Espinoza CG, Richman AV, Azar HA: Carcinomas of the lung: an ultrastructural and immunocytochemical study. American Journal of Clinical Pathology 80:6-13,1983.
11. McDowell EM, Wilson TS, Trump BF: Atypical endocrine tumors of the lung. Archives of Pathology & Laboratory Medicine 105:20-28,1981.

12. Sheppard MN, Corrin B, Bennett MH, Marangos PJ, Bloom SR, Polak JM: Immunocytochemical localization of neuron specific enolase (NSE) in small cell carcinomas and carcinoid tumours of the lung. Histopathology 8,171-181,1984.
13. Vinores SA, Bonnin JM, Rubinstein LJ, Marangos PJ: Immunohistochemical demonstration of neuron-specific enolase in neoplasms of the CNS and other tissues, Archives of Pathology & Laboratory Medicine 108:536-540, 1984.
14. Rode J, Dhillon AP, Dhillon DP, Moss E, Thompson RJ, Spiro SG, Corrin B: Neuroendocrine differentiation in carcinoma of the lung. Journal of Pathology(in press)
15. Lamb D, Krajewski AS, Maloney DJL: Atypical carcinoid tumours of lung: histological features and response with neurone specific enolase technique. Journal of Pathology (in press)
16. Godwin JD: Carcinoid tumours. An analysis of 2837 cases. Cancer 36: 560-569.
17. Huhti E,Sutinen S, Saloheimo M: Survival among patients with lung cancer An epidemiologic study. American Review Respiratory Disease 124:13-16, 1981.
18. Arrigoni MG, Woolner LB, Bernatz PE: Atypical carcinoid tumours of the lung. Journal of Thoracic & Cardiovascular Surgery 64:413-421,1972.
19. Mills SE, Cooper PH, Walker AN, Kron IL: Atypical carcinoid tumour of the lung: a clinicopathological study of 17 cases. American Journal of Surgical Pathology 6:543-654,1982.
20. Gould VE, Linnoila RI, Memoli VA, Warren WH: Neuroendocrine components of the bronchopulmonary tract: hyperplasia, dysplasias and neoplasms. Laboratory Investigation 49:519-537,1983.
21. Jones RA, Dawson IMP: Morphology and staining patterns of endocrine tumours in the gut, pancreas and bronchus and their possible significance. Histopathology 1:137-150,1977.
22. Wise WS, Bonder D, Aikawa M, Hsieh CL: Carcinoid tumour of the lung with varied histology. American Journal of Surgical Pathology 6:261-267,1982.
23. Becker NH, Soifer I: Benign clear cell tumor ("sugar tumor") of lung. Cancer 27:712-719,1971.
24. Walter P, Warter A, Morand G: Carcinoids oncocytaire bronchique. Etude histologique, histochimique et ultrastructurale. Virchows Archives , Pathology Anatomy and Histology 379:85-97,1978.
25. Sklar JL, Churg A, Bencsch KG: Oncocytic carcinoid tumor of the lung. American Journal of Surgical Pathology 4:287-292,1980.
26. Scharifker D, Marchevsky A: Oncocytic carcinoid of lung: an ultra-structural analysis. Cancer 47:530 532,1981.
27. Salyer DC, Salyer WR, Eggleston JC: Bronchial carcinoid tumours. Cancer 36:1522-1537,1975.
28. Ranchod M, Levine GD: Spindle-cell carcinoid tumours of the lung. A clinicopathologic study of 35 cases. American Journal Surgical Pathology 4:315-331,1980.

ADDITIONAL NOTE AND REFERENCES

McCaughan et al (1985) report 124 bronchial carcinoids:factors predisposing to recurrence were tumour size greater than 3 cm, atypical carcinoid histology and lymph node metastases. Paladugu et al (1985) recommend the terms KCC-I, -II and -III instead of the typical carcinoids and small cell cancers respectively. At presentation all their KCC-I were stage I tumours but only 61% of KCC-II. KC-I and -II tumours measured 1.5 and 2.8 cm mean diameter and had a mortality of 1.7% and 27%, respectively.

29. McCaughan BC, Martini N, Baines MS: Bronchial carcinoids. Journal Thoracic Cardiovascular Surgery 89:8-17,1985.
30. Paladugu RR, Benfield JR, Pak HY, Moss RK, Teplitz L: Broncho-pulmonary Kulchitzky cell carcinomas: a new classification scheme for typical and atypical carcinoids. Cancer 55:1303-1311,1985

INTRA- AND INTEROBSERVER PROBLEMS IN THE HISTOPATHOLOGIC CLASSIFICATION
OF MALIGNANT LUNG TUMORS

FRED R.HIRSCH

1. INTRODUCTION

During the last decade an increased focusing on the histopathologic
classification of lung cancer has developed. This has been prompted by
the fact that the treatment modality and prognosis for some patients
was strongly dependent on the histopathologic classification. In order
to give the patient appropriate treatment - chemotherapy or not - a
strict separation of small cell and non-small cell lung cancer was de-
manded. During the same time the biological research activities in lung
cancer have expanded, and pathologists have characterized the experimental material (i.e. tissue cultures and nude mice tumors) as well.

An increased amount of therapeutic and histopathologic studies have
accompanied multiple national and international cooperative studies on
lung cancer. However, in order to have a reliable comparison of the
studies fron one institution to another an exact and reproducible histopathologic classification is mandatory.

2. WHO-CLASSIFICATION

The first attempt to make an international classification of lung
tumors was done in 1958 by the World Health Organization (WHO) (1). The
tentative WHO classification from 1958 was adapted by the Veterans Administration Lung Cancer Study Group (VALG) and was tested in more than
2000 surgically removed specimens (2). They found the overall classification practical, but demonstrated inconsistent criteria for identification of certain tumors, which will be described below.

In 1965, the WHO reconvened the pathology committee and in 1967 the
first official classification of lung tumors was published (3). However,
still discrepancy in the criteria and nomenclature was observed. In 1971
a Working Party for Therapy of Lung Cancer (WP-L) was established in the
United States. The Pathologists in this group deviced a classification
of malignant lung tumors compatible with the WHO-classification as well
as the VALG classification (4).

After ten years of experience with the first classification, WHO
revised the classification of lung tumors in 1977 and published in 1981
(5). At the meeting in Geneva 1977 on the histologic classification of
lung tumors 16 pathologists from 12 different countries assembled to
agree upon an international classification of lung tumors. Some basic
principles were followed: The classification should be acceptable and
useful in every histopathologic department throughout the world. Therefore, the classification was based on simple light microscopic findings,
using routine staining methods, which sould be available in all laboratories i.e. hematoxylin-eosin, mucin- and keratin stains.

3. INTRAOBSERVER PROBLEMS

In 1970 Feinstein et al. focused on the intraobserver problems in the diagnosis of lung cancer (6). Five experienced pathologists gave two independent readings of 50 different specimens. Significant disagreement between the first and second reading of the same slide by the same pathologist occurred in a range of 2 percent for the most consistent reader and 20 percent for the least consistent. Most problems concerned the poorly differentiated tumors. No other studies have been published concerning the intraobserver variability of the lung cancer classification in general. The intraobserver variation of the WHO-subclassification of small cell carcinoma has been examined by Hirsch (7). The examination was based on two independent readings of 100 slides. The diagnostic reproducibility of morphologic subtyping small cell carcinoma was about 90%. However, the study was undertaken by a person specially trained for classifying these particular tumors. The question of whether a similar high reproducibility could be obtained by the individual pathologist in the diagnostic routine has yet to be solved.

4. INTEROBSERVER PROBLEMS

Using the first tentative WHO classification of lung tumors, Yesner et al. drew attention to the difficulty of obtaining consistency among different observers in the diagnosis of malignant lung tumors (2). The unanimity among 3 experienced panelists in the latter study was very low with regard to poorly differentiated carcinoma in general. Unanimity in the diagnosis of large-cell carcinoma was only obtained in 10% of more than 400 slides. For small cell carcinoma unanimity was observed in 34% of the cases of "polygonal" subtype verus 84% for the classical "oat-cell". For poorly differentiated adenocarcinoma and squamous cell carcinoma unanimity was obtained in 43-47%. Similar findings were reported in a later study by Feinstein et al. (6). Disagreement of five observers from the consensus reading was 2-5% for well differentiated adeno- and squamous cell carcinomas, 23-25% for undifferentiated adeno- and squamous cell carcinomas and 40-42% for poorly differentiated squamous cell- and adenocarcinomas.Stanley and Matthews reported in an interobserver analysis a relative high diagnostic agreement for small cell carcinoma (89%) and squamous cell carcinoma (86%), but a low agreement was obtained for the initial diagnosis of large cell carcinoma (40%). For an initial large-cell carcinoma was adenocarcinoma (23%) and squamous cell carcinoma (22%) (8).

Using the current WHO classification an interobserver variability study was performed on the subclassification of small°cell carcinoma (9). Unanimity among 3 panelists in the diagnosis of small cell carcinoma as the main cell type was obtained in 94% of 93 histologic slides. It was concluded that the criteria used for small cell carcinoma as a distinct histopathologic entity were reproducible among different pathologists. However, the aim of the latter study was not primarily to evaluate the criteria for small cell carcinoma as an entity, but to evaluate the reproducibility of the WHO subtyping of this disease. Therefore, the material was selected in such a way that all the slides examined were diagnosed as small cell carcinoma primarily by one of the panelists, and not a consecutive study of a large number of several lung tumors. Unanimity in the diagnoses was obtained in 54% of the slides. An especially poor consistency was observed in the interpretation of the tumors containing morphologic features of mixed small cell/large cell carcinoma. As a consequence of the latter study the morphologic criteria have been discussed by the authors and more recently in the pathology group of "International Association for the Study of Lung Cancer", and a change in the concept and terminology of small cell carcinoma has been recommended (10).

5. CYTOLOGY

With regard to cytologic classification of malignant tumors several studies have shown a good correlation between the cytological diagnosis when performed by the experienced cytologists, and the histopathologic examination. This is observed especially for the well differentiated squamous cell- and adenocarcinoma and small cell carcinoma, with a diagnostic specificity of cell typing in about 90-100% (11, 12). However, intra- or interobserver studies in the cytopathologic classification of malignant lung tumors are sparse in the literature. In a study of diagnostic reproducibility of transthoracic aspiration biopsy an intraobserver correlation of 90-100% in cell typing was observed for the experienced pathologist. Discrepancies were seen between two investigators in nearly all of the major histologic types, but these were in none of the cases statistically significant (13).

6. COMMENTS AND FUTURE PROSPECTS

Before a new histopathologic classification is introduced into routine pathology it should ideally be tested by double readings for its consistency. Different pathologists - not only "experts" should be able to reproduce the diagnosis. The clinical relevance should be clearly proven.

The introduction of new techniques producing very small amount of cells or tissue call for a systematic effort for testing the diagnostic reliability of the cyto- and histopathologic classification.

Future studies of the reliability of the histopathologic classification of malignant lung tumors should be encouraged through the mechanisms of slide circulation, workshops and other panel discussions preferably on an international basis and initiated by the scientific organizations.

More technically advanced diagnostic methods i.e. electron microscopy, immuncytochemistry and flow cytometry, might in the future contribute to a more reliable diagnostic classification. However, as these procedures are not available in all the laboratories throughout the world, they should not yet be included in the international classification of tumors designed for routine pathology.

REFERENCES

1. Kreyberg L: Histological Lung Cancer Types. Acta Pathol Microbiol Scand suppl 157,1962
2. Yesner R, Gerstl B and Auerbach O: Application of the World Health Organization Classification of Lung Carcinoma to Biopsy Material. Ann Thorac Surg 1:33-49,1965.
3. Kreyberg L: Histological Typing of Lung Tumors. International Histological Classification of Tumors. Geneva, World Helath Organization, 1967.
4. Matthews MJ: Morphologic Classification of Bronchogenic Carcinoma. Cancer Chem Rep 4:299-301,1973.
5. World Health Organization: Histological Typing of Lung Tumors. 2.Edition. International Histological Classification of Tumors, No.1,Geneva, 1981.

6. Feinstein AR, Gelfman NA and Yesner R: Observer Variability in the Histopathologic Diagnosis of Lung Cancer. Am Rev Resp Dis 101:671-684, 1970.
7. Hirsch FR: Histopathologic Classification and Metastatic Pattern of Small Cell Carcinoma of the Lung. - With Special Reference to the Clinical Implication. Munksgaard, Copenhagen, 1983.
8. Stanley KE and Matthews MJ: Analysis of a Pathology Review of Patients with Lung Tumors. J NCI 66:989-992,1981.
9. Hirsch FR, Matthews MJ and Yesner R: Histopathologic Classification of Small Cell Carcinoma of the Lung - Comments Based on an Interobserver Examination. Cancer 50:1360-1366,1982.
10. Yesner R: Classification of Lung Cancer Histology. N Engl J Med 312: 652-653,1985 (Letter).
11. Kanhouwa SB and Matthews MJ: Reliability of Cytologic Typing of Lung Cancer. Acta Cytol 20:229-232,1976.
12. Frozan YS and Frost JK: Cytopathologic Diagnosis of Lung CAncer. In: Straus MJ (ed): "Lung Cancer. Clinical Diagnosis and Treatment". Second Edition. Grune & Stratton, New York,1983,pp 113-125.
13. Francis D and Højgaard K: Transthoracic Aspiration Biopsy. A Study of Diagnostic Reproducibility. Acta Path Microbiol Scand A85:889-896,1977.

DIFFERENTIAL DIAGNOSIS OF METASTATIC LESIONS IN THE LUNG.

D.J. Ruiter

1.INTRODUCTION

Focal lung lesions may consist of tumor-like conditions,primary benign tumors, primary malignant tumors or tumor metastases. Tumor-like conditions that may mimic primary lung cancer or metastatic cancer in the lung not only radiologically but also histologically are reactive lesions like plasma cell granuloma, sugar tumor, sclerosing hemangioma, and hamartomas (1). A single focal lesion in the lung is more likely to be primary than secondary lung cancer (2). However, a solitary lung metastasis may be seen in patients with primary tumors of the breast, uterus, testis, colon, kidney and urinary bladder, and in malignant melanoma (2). The carcinomas with the highest propensity to produce metastatic lung disease are those arising in the lung, the breast, the gastrointestinal tract, and the genitourinary system (2). Discrete hematogenous metastatic lung nodules may be found in malignant melanomas, bone sarcomas, trophoblastic tumors and renal cell and thyroid carcinoma (2). Diffuse interstitial and lymphangitic infiltration is found in tumors of the liver, pancreas, stomach, and breast (2). Cytological or histological diagnosis can be obtained by bronchoscopy, bronchial brushing, mediastinoscopy, percutaneous needle aspiration, and percutaneous trephine lung biopsy (2). In the following paragraphs principles and practice of pathological diagnosis of metastatic tumors will be discussed and relevant examples will be given.

2.PRINCIPLES OF PATHOLOGICAL DIAGNOSIS

The assessment of the tumor type and the estimation of the origin of the tumor (i.e. the site of the primary tumor) are the major issues addressed to the pathologist. Thorough gross examination of pulmonary specimens resected for neoplastic disease (3) may indicate a topological association with a pre-existing structure, which helps the pathologist in making a diagnosis of primary lung cancer (4).

Assessment of the tumor type is based on the recognition of signs of differentiation in the tumor cells. In well- and moderately differentiated tumors in most cases the tumor type can be assessed employing conventional light microscopy on paraffin sections only. However, in poorly differentiated tumors the detection of subtle differentiation products often necessitates the use of additional techniques, such as immunohistochemistry and electron microscopy (5-8). These differentiation products include membrane determinants (e.g. immune globulins, certain glycoproteins, desmosomes, microvilli), cytoskeletal proteins especially of the intermediate size (9, 10) (i.e. cytokeratins, vimentin, desmin, neurofilament) and other cytoplasmic determinants (e.g. enzymes, hormones, immune globulins, pigments, (neuro-) secretory granules). Often the application of additional techniques will improve or refine the diagnosis. In any case it is very important to identify or exclude drug-responsive cancers, such as lymphoma, carcinomas of breast, prostate or thyroid, and testicular tumors (11).

The estimation of the origin of the primary tumor is mainly based on the assessment of the tumor type in combination with knowledge about the possible sites of origin and the distribution of metastases from various tumor types. A pulmonary metastatic lesions having the appearance of squamous cell carcinoma is most likely derived from a primary tumor in the lung, nose-throat region or uterine cervix in a female patient. In a metastatic lesion consisting of adenocarcinoma the subtype may give an important clue to the elucidation of the site of the primary tumor. For instance, a papillary adenocarcinoma is probably derived from the thyroid, ovary, kidney or lung. In addition to the assessment of the tumor type the identification of tumor-origin related determinants (12) using immunohistochemistry or in some instances enzyme histochemistry, is important. Highly specific markers in this respect are prostate-specific acid phosphatase and thyreoglobulin; also the determination of cytokeratin subtypes may be informative (13). Less specific markers include carcino embryonal antigen (14), milk fat globulin, and the estrogen receptor.

3. PRACTICAL ASPECTS

The pathological diagnosis of cancer is based on gross examination and conventional histology using paraffin sections. However, in an increasing proportion of cases additional techniques are necessary to confirm, refine or establish the diagnosis. For optimal application of these techniques different fixation procedures are required (Table 1). Therefore, it is very important that <u>unfixed</u> biopsy specimens are submitted directly to the pathologist. If there is any doubt about the representivity of a biopsy specimen frozen section examination should be performed so that the biopsy can be repeated immediately if necessary.

Table 1.

<u>Diagnostic work-up</u> (1)

Incisional or excisional biopsy:

      fresh, unfixed tissue transport immediately to

      PATHOLOGY LABORATORY

      1. formalin fixation for conventional histology

      2. snap freeze, store at -70°C for
         immuno-histochemistry

      3. glutaraldehyde for electron microscopy

      4. imprint preparation for cytology

Additional techniques should be employed step-wise, based on the histological differential diagnosis (Table 2). Information provided by

Table 2.

<u>Diagnostic work-up</u> (2)

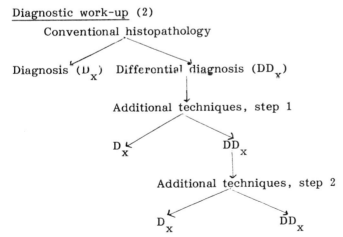

these techniques should be incorporated into the pathological diagnosis and not reported separately by technique specialists. It is the challenge to the pathologist to seek the specific diagnosis with the least possible amount of time, injury and expense to the patient.

In a poorly differentiated malignant tumor the differential diagnosis includes carcinoma, sarcoma, lymphoma and melanoma. Immunohistochemistry and electron microscopy identifying certain differentiation products will help to discriminate between these possibilities (Table 3). Expression of cytokeratin only will indiciate carcinoma. Co-expression of cytokeratin and vimentin or cytokeratin and neurofilament may be found in certain carcinomas (15, 16) (renal cell carcinoma, neuroendocrine carcinoma of the skin) and certain sarcomas (17, 18) (synovial sarcoma, epitheloid sarcoma). It is also found in carcinosarcoma and teratoma. Subtyping of carcinoma can be performed in further steps. Leio- and rhabdomyosarcoma will show expression of desmin. In most other types of sarcoma vimentin is the only filament protein expressed. Further immunohistochemical and electronmicroscopical study is needed to refine the diagnosis. Malignant lymphoma is characterized by the presence of common leukocyte antigen and vimentin. Identification of B cell, T cell or histiocytic differentiation products must be performed for further classification. Although monoclonal antibodies are very sensitive to detect melanoma-associated antigens their diagnostic specificity is not sufficient (19). Therefore, electron microscopy should be performed in order to demonstrate melanosomes, the organels that are involved in melanin synthesis.

Table 3.

Diagnostic work-up (3)

Conventional histopathology shows a poorly differentiated malignant tumor.

Therefore, application of special techniques is necessary.

step 1   The differential
                                                diagnosis includes:

	Differentiation products	CA	SA	LY	MEL
	cytokeratin		+	-(+) -	-
	vimentin		-(+)	+	+	+
IH	desmin		-	-,+	-	-
	neurofilament		-(+)	-	-	-
	common leukocyte antigen		-	-	+	-
	melanoma-associated antigens		-(+)	-	-	+
EM	desmosomes		+	-(+) -	±
	melanosomes		-	-	-	+

Step 2 or more depends on the results of step 1.

IH = immunohistochemistry   CA= carcinoma LY= lymphoma
EM = electron microscopy   SA= sarcoma   MEL= melanoma

CONCLUSIONS.

- For optimal diagnosis of metastatic tumors in the lung fresh unfixed tissue should be submitted immediately to the pathologist.
- The basis of pathological diagnosis of cancer is gross examination and conventional histology; special additional diagnostic techniques should be applied step-wise guided by the histopathological differential diagnosis.
- Information provided by special techniques should be incorporated into the pathological diagnosis and not reported separately.
- In cases of metastasis of unknown origin the diagnostic approach must be directed towards the identification or exclusion of drug-responsive tumors.

REFERENCES.

1. Katzenstein AL, Purvis Jr, R, Gmelich J, Askin F: Pulmonary resection for metastatic renal adenocarcinoma. Pathologic findings and therapeutic value. Cancer 41: 712-23, 1978.

2. Schwaber JR: Diagnostic approaches in metastatic lung disease. Med. Clin. North Am. 59: 277-283, 1975.

3. Carter D: Pathologic examination of major pulmonary specimens resected for neoplastic disease. Pathol. Annual 18: 315-332, 1983 (part 2).

4. Bakris GL, Mulopulos GP, Korchik R, Ezdinli EZ, Ro J, Yoon B-H: Pulmonary scar carcinoma. A clinicopathologic analysis. Cancer 52: 493-7, 1983.

5. Azar HA, Espinoza CG, Richman AV, Saba SR, Wang T: "Undifferentiated" large cell malignancies: An ultrastructural and immunocytochemical study. Human Pathol. 13: 323-33, 1982.

6. Mackay B, Ordonez NG: The role of the pathologist in the evaluation of poorly differentiated tumors. Seminars Oncol. 9: 396-415, 1982.

7. Fleuren GJ, Ruiter DJ, Warnaar SO: Het gebruik van antilichamen in de diagnostiek van kanker. Medisch Jaar 1984, Bohn Scheltema, Holkema, Amsterdam.

8. Ghadially FN: The role of electron microscopy in the determination of tumor histogenesis. Diagn. Histopathol. 4: 245-62, 1981.

9. Osborn M, Weber K: Biology of disease: Tumor diagnosis by intermediate filament typing: A novel tool for surgical pathology. Lab. Invest. 48: 372-94, 1983.

10. Ramaekers FCS, Puts J. Kant A. Moesker O, Jap P, Vooys P: Differential diagnosis of human carcinomas, sarcomas and their metastases using antibodies to intermediate-sized filaments. Eur. J. Cancer Clin. Oncol. 18: 1251-7, 1982.

11. Hobbs J, Rodriguez AR: Metastatic cancer of unknown primary site. Am. Fam. Physician 22: 164-6, 1980.

12. Damjanov I, Knowles BB: Monoclonal antibodies and tumor-associated antigens. Lab. Invest. 48: 510-25, 1983.

13. Moll R, Franke WW, Schiller DL, Geiger B, Krepler R: The catalog of human cytokeratins: pattern of expression in normal epithelia, tumors and cultured cells. Cell 31: 11-24, 1982.

14. Nap M, Ten Hoor KA, Fleuren GJ: Cross-reactivity with normal antigens in commercial anti-CEA sera used for immunohistology. The need for tissue controls and absorptions. Am. J. Clin. Pathol. 79: 25-31, 1983.

15. Herman CJ, Moesker O, Kant A, Ramaekers FCS. Is renal cell (Grawitz) tumor a carcinosarcoma? Evidence from analysis of intermediate filament types. Virchows Arch (Cell Pathol) 44: 73-79, 1983.

16. Van Muyen GNP, Ruiter DJ, Warnaar SO. Intermediate filaments in Merkel cell tumors. Human Pathol. 1985, in press.

17. Miettinen M, Lehto V-P., Virtanen I. Keratin in the epithelial-like cells of classical biphasic synovial sarcoma. Virchows Arch (Cell Pathol) 40: 157-161, 1982.

18. Miettinen M, Lehto V-P, Vartio T, Virtanen I. Epitheloid sarcoma. Ultrastructural and immunohistochemical features suggesting synovial origin Arch Pathol. Lab. Med. 106: 620-623, 1982.

19. Van Duinen SG, Ruiter DJ, Hageman Ph., Vennegoor C, Dickersin GR, Scheffer E, Rümke Ph.: Immunohistochemical and histochemical tools in the diagnosis of amelanotic melanoma. Cancer 53: 1566-1573, 1984.

CYTOLOGY AND LUNG CANCER

WILLIAM W. JOHNSTON

1. INTRODUCTION

It is now generally accepted in just about every medical care facility throughout the world that clinical cytology has a premier role to play in the diagnosis of lung cancer. Duke University was among those several medical institutions who first recognized the potential impact of exfoliative cytology on clinical medicine. Only three years after the publication of the now famous Papanicolaou and Traut monograph in 1943, the Duke University Department of Obstetrics and Gynecology had established a laboratory of clinical cytology for the diagnosis of cancers of the female genital tract. During the decade of the 1950's, cytological examinations of sputum, bronchial washings, and other specimens were gradually introduced. Through this author's own investigations in respiratory cytology spanning a period of a quarter of a century, he has attempted to measure both qualitatively and quantitatively the validity of the cytological method in lung cancer diagnosis (4,7-16,20).

In one large series of lung cancer patients studied, it was found that a cytological diagnosis of unequivocal cancer had been established in 50% of these patients. One specimen only of sputum had established a cancer diagnosis of 27% of patients had one bronchial wash or brush in 22%. No significant difference was found in diagnostic significance between bronchial washings and bronchial brushings. When at least five satisfactory specimens were examined consisting of any combination of sputum and bronchial material, a cytological diagnosis of cancer had been established in 87% of lung cancer patients. Furthermore, these specimens had achieved an accuracy level of nearly 96% in being able to differentiate between small cell cancers and "non-small cell" cancers, a distinction on which the clinical oncologist had been able to base therapeutic decisions (9,11,13).

Even more recently, cytology of the respiratory tract has been revolutionized by a combination of two factors: the maturation of a high degree of sophistication in radiological technology, making possible the precise vizualization and localization of masses in the lungs, and the reintroduction of a technique of sampling of such vizualized lesions by the insertion into them of a fine bore needle (1,3-4,10,16,18-19). The remainder of this discussion will concentrate on the chronicle of the development of fine needle aspiration biopsy (FNAB) at one institution.

The general technque of FNAB came into use at Duke University Medical Center in the early 1970's. At the end of the year 1984, the files of the cytopathology laboratory recorded a total of 5060 aspirates examined, 30% were from lung.

In our current procedure, any patient found to have a demonstrable radiographical abnormality in the lung fields is a potential candidate for FNAB. A further decision on whether or not to proceed with the aspiration is based upon the level of suspicion that the visualized nodule or density represents a cancer or an infectious process and on the morphological evidence provided by prior cytological and histological specimens obtained from the respiratory tract. All aspirations are performed by a radiologist using fluoroscopy or computerized axial tomography. A 22 gauge Chiba needle with a 20 ml. syringe is inserted percutaneously into the lung mass. From the aspirate two direct smears are prepared for immediate wet fixation in 95% ethanol and staining with the Papanicolaou method. The remaining aspirate is then mixed with 10 ml. balanced salts solution and brought to the laboratory for further procedures. Aliquots of this cellular suspension are processed for membrane filters, direct smears, cytocentrifuge specimens, and cell blocks. Since 1978 the principle of immediate consultation has been practiced by which fixed smears are stained by a rapid Papanicolaou staining technique and unfixed cellular suspensions are stained with a 4% aqueous solution of toluidine blue. By this procedure the radiologist can be given an immediate assessment of the cellular content of the aspirate and therefore an implied assessment of whether or not it is satisfactory for diagnosis. If it is determined to be unsatisfactory, the aspiration is repeated immediately. All of the cellular preparations are screened by cytotechnologists and are then referred to a cytopathologist for final diagnostic interpretation.

The following table records a division of the patients sampled through December, 1984 into the major diagnostic categories of primary lung cancer; cancer metastatic to the lung; inconclusive diagnoses; and benign diagnoses:

DIAGNOSTIC CATEGORY	NUMBER PATIENTS	PER CENT PATIENTS
Primary Lung Cancer	653	43.5
Metastatic Cancer	199	13.2
Inconclusive	82	5.5
Benign	568	37.8
Total	1502	100.0

In 43.5% of the total patient group, a diagnosis of a primary lung cancer was made; in 13.2% a cancer metastatic to the lung; in 37.8% a benign diagnosis. In 5.5% of patients, cancer was suspected but could not be conclusively diagnosed, by cytological diagnoses alone.

2.PRIMARY LUNG CANCER

In 653 patients, FNAB's of the lungs were interpreted as being conclusively diagnostic for a primary malignant neoplasm. These neoplasms shown in the following table have been divided according to their histological type:

DIAGNOSTIC CATEGORY	NUMBER PATIENTS	PER CENT PATIENTS
Squamous Cell Carcinoma	246	37.7
Adenocarcinoma	86	13.2
Large Cell Undifferentiated Carcinoma	193	30.0
Small Cell Undifferentiated Carcinoma	76	11.6
Adenosquamous Carcinoma	23	3.5
Plasmacytoma	2	0.3
Carcinoid	2	0.3
Unclassified	25	3.8
Total	653	100.0

Squamous cell carcinoma was the most frequent diagnosis and was made in 37.7% of patients. The other diagnoses in descending order of frequency were large cell undifferentiated carcinoma, 30.0%; adenocarcinoma, 13.2%; small cell undifferentiated carcinoma 11.6%, and adenosquamous carcinoma 3.5%. In 3.8% of patients, while it was concluded that neoplastic cells were present, no opinion could be reached with respect to their further classification.

There were 122 patients whose cytological diagnoses of primary malignant neoplasm of the lung had been followed within a period of seven days by open thoracotomy or biopsy performed for the purpose of confirming the FNAB diagnosis and carrying out therapeutic resection. This series of patients as tabulated below provided a useful vehicle for correlating cytological and histological interpretations on the same patients:

CYTOLOGICAL DIAGNOSIS	HISTOLOGICAL DIAGNOSIS					
	SCC	AC	LCUC	SCUC	ASC	Carc.
SCC	31	8	2	1	1	0
AC	1	21	0	0	0	0
LCUC	5	18	9	0	0	0
SCUC	1	0	0	10	0	0
ASC	0	6	0	0	2	0
Carc.	0	0	0	0	0	1
Unclassified	0	2	2	0	0	1

SCC = squamous cell carcinoma; AC = adenocarcinoma; LCUC = large cell undifferentiated carcinoma; SCUC = small cell undifferentiated carcinoma; ASC = adenosquamous carcinoma; Carc. = carcinoid.

Cytological diagnoses of squamous cell carcinoma with varying degrees of differentiation had been made in 43 patients. Histological diagnoses of squamous cell carcinoma had been made in 31 of the 43 patients (72%). In eight of the 43, histological diagnoses of adenocarcinoma had been made (19%). In a smaller number of patients histological diagnoses of large cell undifferentiated carcinoma (two patients), small cell undifferentiated carcinoma (one patient), and adenosquamous carcinoma had been made. Among 22 patients whose FNAB had been interpreted as adenocarcinoma, 21 (95%) had also been recognized as adenocarcinoma. The tissue from one patient had been histologically diagnosed as squamous cell carcinoma. There were 32 patients in whom a FNAB diagnosis of large cell undifferentiated carcinoma had been rendered. Tissue from nine patients (28%) had also been given this diagnosis on histology. But 18 of the 32 patients (56%) and 5 of the 32 (16%) were shown on histological examination to have adenocarcinomas and squamous cell carcinomas respectively. No small cell cancers were recognized histologically in this group. Among the eleven patients with cytological diagnoses of small cell undifferentiated carcinoma, ten were also shown by histological examination to have a small cell cancer. In one patient the histological diagnosis of squamous cell carcinoma undoubtedly reflected either a squamous cancer component arising in small cell undifferentiated carcinoma or another lung primary cancer.

In a recent parallel study, the author reviewed all histopathologically confirmed primary lung cancers seen during a recent ten year period. Among the 1117 patients in the group, the division by histological classification was as follows: squamous cell carcinoma 41.4%; adenocarcinoma 27.1%; large cell undifferentiated carcinoma 19.4%; small cell undifferentiated carcinoma 10.9%; and adenosquamous carcinoma

1.2%. In comparing the percentage distribution between the FNAB patient group and the 1117 patients from the histological survey, the percentages of patients with squamous cell carcinoma, small cell carcinoma, and adenosquamous carcinoma are quite similar, but there are significant differences in adenocarcinoma and large cell carcinoma. Some explanation for this discrepancy is documented by a frequent failure of the FNAB specimen to permit a correct recognition of adenomatous differentiation and thus resulting in an assignment of the neoplasm to the classification of large cell undifferentiated carcinoma. Furthermore, a number of additional reasons can be cited for these varying levels of correlation between the cytological and histological interpretation on the same lung tumor. Perhaps the most telling factor of all is the current growing general awareness of the cellular pleomorphism present in most of the "non-small cell" bronchogenic carcinomas. Recent studies in the literature suggest that the large cell carcinomas and poorly differentiated carcinomas, whether of adenomatous or squamous differentiation, may show on ultrastructural examination patterns which are dualistic or even triadic in differentiation. Hess et al. in a series of studies on the histogenesis of lung cancer have shown that many poorly to well-differentiated squamous cell carcinomas, poorly to well-differentiated adenocarcinomas, and giant cell carcinomas, diagnosed as such by conventional light microscopic criteria, were in reality tumors exhibiting dual differentiation toward both squamous cell carcinoma and adenocarcinoma (5). Horie and Ohta examined by light and electron microscopy 26 human lung tumors classified as large cell undifferentiated carcinomas. On the basis of their observations, these investigators were able to subclassify all of these tumors into squamous, adenosquamous, and giant cell (6). Dingemans and Mooi investigated by electron microscopy a series of 40 lung tumors which had been diagnosed by conventional light microscopy as squamous cell carcinoma. Both at the tissue and at the cellular level the tumors showed highly variable ultrastructural details embracing both tonofibrils and desmosomes on one hand and unmistakable adenomatous differentiation on the other (2). From such studies as these, one is tempted to conclude that the major proportion of the "non-small cell" carcinomas of the lung are in reality adenosquamous carcinomas. Such a possibility would well account for the discrepancies that one encounters in the various cited summaries of cyto-histological correlations. It is worthy of emphasis, however, that the ability on the FNAB specimen to distinguish between the small cell cancers and the "non-small cell" cancers is quite high. In only 2 cases out of the 122 studied by the author was there an apparent non-correlation. This agreement level of 98.4% surpasses that as published by the author several years ago of a 95.5% level of cyto-histological correlation between specimens of sputum and bronchial material and tissues (12). In no instances did the FNAB predict falsely the presence of small cell undifferentiated carcinoma when the lesion was in fact a carcinoid, atypical carcinoid, or lymphoma.

3.SPUTUM,BRONCHIAL MATERIAL AND FNAB

Among the 653 patients with FNAB diagnoses of primary lung cancer in this series, 333 had also been evaluated with specimens of sputum and bronchial material. 163 out of the 333 (48.9%) had had at least one satisfactory sputum or specimen of bronchial material submitted for cytological evaluation. These studies are shown in the following table:

DIAGNOSTIC CATEGORY	FNAB PATIENTS WITH SPUTUM/BRONCHIAL MATERIAL	SUSPICIOUS	POSITIVE
SCC	62	11	19
AC	15	1	6
LCUC	60	10	14
SCUC	15	2	4
ASC	5	3	2
Unclassified	6	1	1
Total	163	28	46

In 74 patients or 45.4% of the 163 so examined, there were cytological changes either conclusively diagnostic (46 patients) or highly suspicious (28 patients) for a malignant neoplasm.

Over the years of its development at DUMC, a formal protocol for FNAB utilization has never been formulated. Individualized physician decisions about the diagnostic approaches to lung lesions have resulted in the data as shown in the table. Information such as this emphasizes yet again the diagnostic effectiveness of conventional respiratory cytological methods. The question then of whether or not FNAB should be the primary diagnostic tool becomes a complex matter of balancing such considerations as length of patient's stay in hospital, other economic factors, the reluctance of some patients to permit their lungs to be pierced by needles, and the morbidity of FNAB. In the experience of our laboratory, sputum and bronchial material provide a high diagnostic yield for lung cancer and in most cases should be used before resorting to FNAB (11).

4. CANCER METASTATIC TO THE LUNG

In the diagnostic assessment with FNAB of a patient with suspected cancer metastatic to the lung, we have approached the problem in the same manner as the surgical pathologist would approach a similar patient. The patient's clinical history is reviewed for either documentation or prior suspicion of a pre-existing neoplasm. All prior histological and cytological specimens are reviewed. Finally, and most significantly, the cellular changes in the FNAB are compared with the pre-existing diagnostic material. The following table summarizes these patients:

TYPE OF NEOPLASM OR TISSUE OF ORIGIN	NUMBER PATIENTS	PER CENT PATIENTS
Malignant Melanoma	51	25.6
Urinary and Male Genital Tract	38	19.1
Breast	26	13.1
Female Genital Tract	30	15.1
Gastro-intestinal Tract	21	10.6
Bone and Soft Tissues	14	7.0
Lymphoma	8	4.0
Mediastinum	3	1.5
Primary Unknown	5	2.5
Salivary Glands	1	0.5
Neuroblastoma	1	0.5
"False Positive"	1	0.5
	199	100.0

70

199 patients were identified with FNAB specimens diagnosed as reflecting cancer metastatic to the lung. This number represents 13.2% of the total patient group of 1502.

With reference to the type of neoplasm, tissue, or organ system of origin, malignant melanoma was seen in 25.6%; neoplasms from the urinary and male genital tract in 19.1%; adenocarcinoma from the breast in 13.1%; neoplasms, usually squamous cell carcinomas, from the female genital tract in 15.1%; adenocarcinoma from the gastrointestinal tract in 10.6%; and neoplasms from the bones and soft tissues in 7.0%. In terms of histological type, the six most common metastatic neoplasms were: malignant melanoma, carcinoma of the breast, adenocarcinoma of the colon, transitional cell carcinoma of the bladder, squamous cell carcinoma of the cervix, and adenocarcinoma of the kidney. The large number of melanomas in this series is accounted for by the existence of a major melanoma treatment clinic at Duke University. FNAB on these patients plays a highly significant role in their therapeutic management.

In this group of patients there was one diagnostic error. The patient was a 58 year old man with a history of a neoplasm of the testis having been resected one year before. He was considered a candidate for FNAB because of a small nodule adjacent to the diaphragm in the left lower lung field. The aspirate was interpreted as containing small numbers of unclassified malignant tumor cells. The nodule was resected and found to be a lipoma with a covering of highly reactive and proliferative mesothelium. On further review of the clinical history, it was found that the patient had never had a testicular neoplasm.

One aspect of the development of FNAB of the lung which has been unusually innovative has been its role in the modification of the diagnostic approach to the patient with prior cancer suspected to be metastatic to the lungs. Before the advent of FNAB, such patients would have been subjected either to thoracotomy or treated on the bases of radiological and clinical findings. In these patients the aspirate will usually reveal the answers to two critical questions: Is the lesion cancerous? If cancerous, is its morphology compatible with that of the primary cancer, or is it a new primary cancer? In patients with multiple primary cancers, an additional answerable question will be: which primary has metastasized?

5. THE EFFECTIVENESS OF FNAB IN THE DETECTION OF MALIGNANT NEOPLASMS OF THE LUNG

In a search for the most objective method for evaluating the accuracy of FNAB in the detection of malignant neoplasms of the lungs, it was elected to compare the FNAB diagnosis in each patient with the histopathological diagnosis revealed upon the excised surgical specimens. For the tissue to qualify in this evaluation, it had to have been the lesion in the lung that was aspirated and to have been resected seven days or less following the aspiration. There were 171 patients in the DUMC series who were found to fulfill these criteria. The results are tabulated as follows:

DIAGNOSTIC CATEGORY	NUMBER PATIENTS	PER CENT PATIENTS
FNAB and Tissue Positive for Cancer	137	80.1
FNAB Negative and Tissue Positive	32	18.7
FNAB Positive and Tissue Negative	2	1.2
TOTAL	171	100.0

In 137 patients or 80.1%, both the FNAB and the histological specimen reflected a diagnosis of cancer. In 32 (18.7%) patients the tissue revealed a cancer which had been missed by the needle aspiration. Re-screening of these specimens failed to reveal tumor cells which may have been overlooked previously. In two patients, one of whom has already been mentioned in the section on metastases, the tissue examination could not sustain the cytological diagnosis. These two cases then are considered to be "false positive" diagnoses for cancer.

This observer experienced some difficulty in arriving at a conclusive method for assessing the effectiveness of FNAB of the lung in the prediction of the presence of a malignant neoplasm. By convention, the reference standard for any cytological method has been histopathology. In the present series, many patients with primary cancers had been treated on the basis of the cytological diagnosis alone. In the patients with suspected metastatic cancer, the FNAB in itself was considered the verification. There were, however, 171 patients noted above from whom tissue had been obtained within a short interval following the aspiration. This group of patients then was used to address the question of effectiveness of detection. This detection rate of 80.1% of malignant neoplasms of the lungs compares favorably with those reported by others (3).

6.FNAB AND NON-NEOPLASTIC LESIONS OF THE LUNG

There were 568 patients in whom no malignant neoplasm was seen and in whom no subsequent studies revealed malignant neoplasm. This patient group was further divided into the following diagnostic categories: negative for cancer and without cellular evidence of inflammation or infectious agent; negative for cancer with nonspecific inflammation; and negative for cancer with evidence of an infectious organism or specific type of inflammatory process. These patients are summarized below:

DIAGNOSTIC CATEGORY		NUMBER PATIENTS	PER CENT PATIENTS
Negative for Cancer and Without Inflammation		439	77.3
Negative For Cancer and Inflammation, Nonspecific		80	14.1
Inflammation, Specific			
Bacteria	7		
Tuberculosis	1		
Nocardiosis	1		
Blastomycosis	3		
Cryptococcosis	5		
Histoplasmosis	3		
Candidiasis	1		
Aspergillosis	7		
Phycomycosis	3		
Granuloma	15		
Abscess	3	49	8.6
		568	100.0

The third category, comprising 49 patients, is of particular interest here, because of the highly specific diagnostic information learned from the FNAB about the patient. In many of those cases in which an infectious organism was identified, it was immediately apparent on the toluidine blue stained specimen. Upon notice of the presence of such an organism, the radiologist would then make a second needle pass into the lung and submit the aspirate for culture.

In two patients, coin lesions called negative by FNAB were shown on resection to be hamartomas.

The author has previously emphasized the importance of cytological methods in the evaluation of patients without lung cancer (7-10,12,14-15). 8.6% of patients in this category benefitted from FNAB diagnosis which either detected an infectious organism or recognized the morphological manifestations of a specific type of inflammation.

7.CONCLUSIONS AND FUTURE DIRECTIONS

Fine needle aspiration biopsy of the lung at Duke University Hospital was introduced to the institution through a cooperative effort between the Imaging Division of Radiology and the Division of Cytopathology. An initial submission of one specimen per year in 1973 swelled to 415 per year in 1984. It is now the most frequently requested FNAB examination. Undoubtedly this is the experience that has begun to unfold in countless hospitals and clinics throughout the world. The literature now contains many studies which have established the effectiveness of FNAB and which have been well summarized in a number of book chapters, monographs, and textbooks (1,3-4,10,16,18-19). Other presentations in this symposium summarize developments in areas such as applications of monoclonal antibodies (MAb s) in imaging and targeting. Active studies in the application of monoclonal antibodies to tumor associated antigens in the diagnostic interpretation of FNAB s are currently in progress in our laboratories in anticipation of the powerful diagnostic, prognostic, and therapeutic tool that could be forged by the combined technologies of the cellular specimen of aspirate and operationally specific monoclonal antibodies raised against tumor associated antigens. The following table presents a brief summary of our laboratory experience in the immunoperoxidase staining of 52 FNAB s from various lung cancers with monoclonal antibody B72.3, an IgG antibody raised by Schlom and associates against a human metastatic breast carcinoma (21). Prior studies by our laboratory had illustrated the usefulness of this antibody in the diagnostic distinction between cancer and reactive mesothelium in effusions (17).

FNAB LUNG TUMOR TYPE	STAINING WITH MAb B72.3	
	NO. POS.	NO. TESTED
Adenocarcinoma	11 (100%)	11
Adenosquamous Carcinoma	7 (100%)	7
Squamous Cell Carcinoma	15 (88%)	17
Large Cell Undifferentiated Carcinoma	4 (40%)	10
Small Cell Undifferentiated Carcinoma	0	7

100% of the adenocarcinomas and adenosquamous carcinomas expressed reactivity with MAb B72.3. A lesser percentage of the squamous cell carcinomas and large cell undifferentiated carcinomas showed some reactivity. In striking contrast, none of the seven FNAB s of small cell undifferentiated carcinoma exhibited any reactivity with MAb B72.3. Neither was any staining with MAb B72.3 noted in benign lung lesions. Studies such as these have been persuasive in convincing this author of the future exciting role that may be played by monoclonal antibodies in the cytological diagnosis of lung cancer.

REFERENCES

1. Bonfiglio T: Transthoracic Thin Needle Aspiration Biopsy. Edited by W.W. Johnston. Masson, Paris, New York, 1983.
2. Dingemans KP, Mooi WJ: Ultrastructure of squamous cell carcinoma of the lung. Pathol Annu; 19 Pt 1:249-273, 1984.
3. Frable WJ: Thin Needle Aspiration Biopsy. WB Saunders, Philadelphia, 1983.
4. Heaston DK, Mills SR, Moore AV, and Johnston WW: "Percutaneous Thoracic Needle Biopsy." In Pulmonary Disease, edited by Charles Putman. Appleton-Century-Crofts, 1981.
5. Hess FG, McDowell EM, Resau JH and Trump BF: The respiratory epithelium: IX. Validity and reproducibility of revised cytologic criteria for human and hamster respiratory tract tumors. Acta Cytol 25:485-498, 1981.
6. Horie A and Ohta M: Ultrastructural features of large cell carcinoma of the lung with reference to the prognosis of patients. Human Pathol 12:423-432, 1981.
7. Johnston WW, Schlein B, and Amatulli J: Cytopathologic Diagnosis of Fungus Infections. Acta Cytol. 13:488-492, 1969.
8. Johnston WW and Amatulli J: The Role of Cytology in the Primary Diagnosis of North American Blastomycosis. Acta Cytol. 14:200-204, 1970.
9. Johnston WW and Frable WJ: Cytopathology of the Respiratory Tract - A Review. Am. J. Path. 84:371-424, 1976.
10. Johnston WW and Frable WJ: Diagnostic Respiratory Cytopathology. Masson, Paris, New York, 1979.
11. Johnston WW and Bossen EH: Ten Years of Respiratory Cytopathology at Duke University Medical Center. I. The Cytopathologic Diagnosis of Lung Cancer During the Years 1970-1974; The Significance of Specimen Number and Type. Acta Cytol. 25:103-107, 1981.
12. Johnston WW, and Bossen EH: Ten Years of Respiratory Cytopathology at Duke University Medical Center. II. A Comparison Between Cytopathology and Histopathology in Typing of Lung Cancer During the Years 1970-1974. Acta Cytol. 25:499-505, 1981.
13. Johnston WW: Ten Years of Respiratory Cytopathology at Duke University Medical Center. III. The Significance of Inconclusive Cytopathologic Diagnoses During the Years 1970-1974. Acta Cytol. 26:759-766, 1982.
14. Johnston WW: "Pulmonary Cytopathology in the Compromised Host". Lung Pathology for the Clinician, edited by S.D. Greenberg. Thieme-Stratton, Inc. New York, 1982.
15. Johnston WW: "The Cytopathology of Opportunistic Infections of the Lungs and Other Body Sites." In Compendium on Cytology, Vol. V, Tutorials of Cytology, Chicago, 1983.
16. Johnston WW: Percutaneous FNAB of the Lung. Acta Cytol. 28:218-224, 1984.
17. Johnston WW, Szpak CA, Lottich SC, Thor A and Schlom J: An adenocarcinoma associated determinant in human effusions: Use of a monoclonal antibody as an immunocytochemical adjuvant to diagnoses. Cancer Res 45:1894-1900, 1985.
18. Kaminsky DB: Applications of Fine Needle Aspiration Biopsy to a Community Hospital. Edited by W.W. Johnston. Masson, Paris, New York. 1981.
19. Koss LG: Diagnostic Cytology and Its Histopathologic Bases. 3rd Edition. J.P. Lippincott. Philadelphia, 1978.
20. Lefer L and Johnston WW: Electron Microscopic Observations of Sputum in Alveolar Cell Carcinoma. Acta Cytol. 20:26-31, 1976.

74

21. Nuti M, Teramoto YA, Mariani-Constanti R, Horan Hand P, Colcher D and Schlom J: A monoclonal antibody (B72.3) defines patterns of distribution of a novel tumor-associated antigen in human mammary carcinoma cell populations. Int J Cancer 29:539-545, 1982.

IMMUNOCYTOCHEMICAL ASSESSMENT OF LUNG TUMORS

FRED T. BOSMAN

1.   INTRODUCTION
     Diagnostic histopathology has shown some rather drastic changes in
the last decennium. One aspect of these changes has been the further
refinement of morphological analysis of   tissues   and   cells   by
electronmicroscopy and quantitative (morphometrical) analysis. Another
aspect has been the introduction of immunocytochemistry in the routine
surgical pathology laboratory. This latter methodology has carried
diagnostic pathology beyond the limitations of descriptive morphology by
adding a dimension of functional analysis. The impact of immunocytochemistry on diagnostic pathology has been enormous and is well
illustrated by the fact that presently in a majority of the original
articles in diagnostic pathology journals the reported findings are to a
significant degree supported by immunocytochemical studies.
     The most impressive achievements of the immunocytochemical approach
to problems in diagnostic pathology have been booked in the area of tumor pathology. With target antigens like oncofetal proteins and cellular
constituents and products, such as intermediate filament proteins,
hormones and enzymes, problems in the classification of   primary
neoplasms, the differentiation between primary and metastatic lesions
and the determination of the primary site of metastases of unknown
origin have been approached with variable success (15). With the
advent of the hybridoma methodology numerous monoclonal antibodies,
purportedly specific for tumors of a certain origin or with a particular
type of differentiation, have been generated. Recently the application
of antibodies specific for the various classes of intermediate filament
cytoskeletal proteins have proven to be powerful tools for tumor
classification.
     Also in the study of pulmonary neoplasms immunocytochemistry has
been extensively applied. In this chapter I will discuss a few relevant
methodological aspects, review the antigens which might be useful for
lung tumor classification and finally evaluate the significance of
marker immunocytochemistry for the solution of problems in   the
histopathological diagnosis of lung cancer.

2.   TECHNIQUES
     Since the original description of direct   immunofluorescence,
around four decades ago, an enormous variety of immunocytochemical
techniques has been developed, most of them multistep indirect methods.
The merits and disadvantages of the most important variants have been
reviewed elsewhere (6) and will not be discussed here. In principle,
there are no major differences in sensitivity between these techniques,
they are all relatively simple to perform and provided that specific

antibodies are used, the tissue is properly processed and the execution is done carefully, they will all yield acceptable and reproducible results.

It is essential, however, to keep in mind that not all commercially available antisera meet equally high standards of specificity. It is clear that many conflicting reports in the literature have resulted from inadequately characterized reagents. Even when well characterized specific antisera are used, antisera from different sources may have different characteristics. For obvious reasons it is virtually impossible to standardize polyclonal antisera for diagnostic use. With the advent of monoclonal antibodies of which theoretically unlimited quantities can be produced, standardization has become an attainable goal. When criteria for the classification of neoplasms are to include immunohistochemically determined characteristics, it is essential that standardized reagents are used.

It is equally important to keep in mind that tissue processing procedures always affect the immunoreactivity of the antigen under unvestigation. In addition many antigens differ in the stability of their immunoreactivity under certain conditions. Basement membrane antigens, for example, lose their immunoreactivity after formalin fixation and paraffin embedding but this can be at least partially restored by pepsin treatment (2). Intermediate filament proteins tend to be preserved slightly better in formalin but their immunoreactivity can be improved by trypsin digestion (39). There is no single fixative which provides satisfactory preservation of all diagnostically relevant antigens. For this reason it is important that all tissue specimens are obtained fresh and that an unfixed sample of tumor tissue is snap frozen and stored at $-70\,^{\circ}C$. Often good immunocytochemical results can be obtained on unfixed or mildly fixed cryostat sections when these techniques fail on routinely processed paraffin sections.

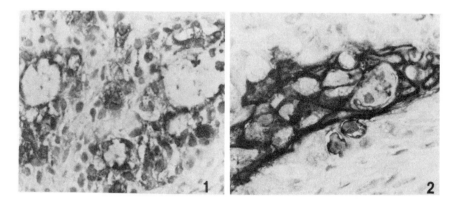

Fig. 1   CEA immunoreactivity in lung adenocarcinoma. Note diffuse cytoplasmic immunoreactivity, more intense surrounding lumena (frozen section; indirect immunoperoxidase, 250 x).

Fig. 2   CEA immunoreactivity in squamous cell lungcarcinoma. The immunoreactivity is confined to an area of keratinization (frozen section; indirect immunoperoxidase, 250 x).

3. ANTIGENS
    A wide variety of biological compounds, which are of potential use
as markers, has been studied in lung tumors. The most important of these
are listed in table I.

TABLE 1. Biological compounds with potential as marker in lung cancer

---

1. oncofetal proteins   –   carcinoembryonic antigen
                             –   pregnancy specific B1 glycoprotein

2. cell products   –   serotonin (5-HT)
                             –   neurohormonal peptides
                             –   chorionic gonadotropin
                             –   surfactant apoprotein

3. cellular constituents   –   enzymes
                                   . neuron specific enolase
                                   . dopa decarboxylase
                                   . histaminase
                                   . creatine kinase B/B
                             –   chromogranin
                             –   epithelial   membrane   antigens   (EMA,
                                  HMFG)
                             –   intermediate filament associated
                                  proteins
                             –   . cytokeratins
                                   . neurofilament proteins
                                   . vimentin
                                   . desmin

4. monoclonal antibody
    defined substances

3.1 Oncofetal proteins
    Of the oncofoetal proteins **carcinoembryonic antigen (CEA)** has been
extensively studied in lung tumors (43, 51). Almost all adenocarcinomas
are CEA-positive and in these tumors almost all cells are positive in a
membrane associated and diffuse cytoplasmic pattern (fig. 1). The large
majority of squamous cell carcinomas is also CEA positive. The
immunoreactivity is usually restricted to areas of keratinization (fig.
2). Also large cell carcinomas and even small cell carcinomas and
carcinoids are often CEA positive.
    CEA has also been extensively studied in mesotheliomas. Most
investigators have reported absence of CEA-immunoreactivity in
mesotheliomas (27, 31, 52, 54) , advocating the use of CEA immunocytochemistry to distinguish between mesothelioma and adenocarcinoma
of the lung. However, a small number of cases of mesothelioma, reactive
with anti-CEA antisera, has been published (3, 12, 18, 22, 43) This
discrepancy may be a result of the use of different antisera as well as
different staining protocols and certainly calls for caution in the use

of CEA immunostaining as the single criterium to differentiate between mesothelioma and primary or metastatic adenocarcinoma.

Pregnancy specific Bl glycoprotein has only been studied occasionally in lung tumors (51). Its frequency of occurrence and also its staining pattern are almost identical to that of CEA. This antigen will therefore not be further discussed.

3.2 Cell products

The respiratory tract contains a complex neuroendocrine system (19) and therefore it is not surprising that endocrine type tumors occur in the lung which, in addition to 5-hydroxytryptamin (5-HT) can produce a variety of **neurohormonal peptides**. Carcinoids, the classical endocrine tumors, frequently produce bombesin, calcitonin and leu-enkephalin (53, 55), peptides which also occur in normal pulmonary neuroepithelial bodies (13). In our own experience (8), more than 50% of these tumors contain 5-HT immunoreactive cells (fig. 3) but only a relatively small proportion shows peptide-hormone immunoreactivity (fig. 4). Atypical carcinoids, which may be an intermediate between classical carcinoids and small cell carcinomas (38), and also small cell carcinomas show peptide hormone production, although less frequent than carcinoids (20).

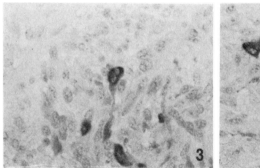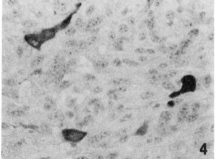

Fig. 3 & 4 5-HT (3) and ACTH (4) immunoreactivity in a lung carcinoid. Only a limited number of cells stain (paraffin section; indirect immunoperoxidase, 250 x).

What is somewhat surprising is that hormone production is by no means restricted to neuroendocrine type tumors but also occurs in adenocarcinomas and large cell carcinomas (24) and even in squamous cell carcinomas (10). This phenomenon probably reflects the existence of multiple lines of differentiation in a tumor (7) and as such is a reflection of the common endodermal derivation of the neuroendocrine and other epithelial cell types of the lung (47).

In addition to those mentioned above, a wide variety of peptides has been detected by immunocytochemistry in carcinoids and small cell carcinomas of the lung (20, 53). There appears to be no specific pattern of neurohormonal peptide immunoreactivity in these tumors. Gastrin releasing peptide (GRP), which is the mammalian analogue of the amphibian peptide bombesin and may be the substance responsible for the bombesin immunoreactivity, is the most frequently detected peptide (20, 45).

Elevated plasma hormone levels occur much more frequently than clinically evident ectopic hormonal syndromes (10), indicating that often tumors produce biologically inactive precursor substances (23). Immunocytochemistry not infrequently fails to detect the site of hormone production in tumors, even when elevated tissue concentrations can be demonstrated by radioimmunoassay (24).

Chorionic gonadotropin is another hormonally active cell product of which elevated plasma levels have been detected in patients with lung cancer (10). Also by immunocytochemistry β-HCG has been detected (51). A recent report on HCG immunolocalization in pancreatic endocrine tumors claims that in these tumors the presence of α-HCG is strongly correlated with malignant behaviour (26). We have found α-HCG in about 25% of a series of lung carcinoids which were all benign, indicating that in these tumors this association does not exist (unpublished observations).

Surfactant-apoprotein has been detected by immunocytochemistry in approximately 50% of bronchiolo-alveolar carcinomas (14) Similar findings are described by Shimosato and Kodama in chapter 3. In these tumors by electron-microscopy the presence of characteristic osmiophilic lamellar bodies could be demonstrated, indicating that they probably originate from type II pneumocytes. Although the use of surfactant-apoprotein as a lung specific marker has not been systematically studied, this antigen may be of help in the differentiation between primary and metastatic bronchiolo-alveolar like adenocarcinomas.

3.3 Cellular constituents.

In former days many attempts have been made to characterize tumors by enzyme-cytochemistry, based on the assumption that there might be tumor-specific patterns of expression. These early attempts, however, were largely unsuccessful. Recent attempts to use immunocytochemical methods for the detection of isozymes, specific for certain cell types, have yielded more promising results. After the discovery of a neuron-specific isozyme of the glycolytic enzyme enolase the finding that this neuron-specific-enolase (NSE) can also be found in neuroendocrine cells throughout the body led to its exploration as a marker for neuroendocrine tumors. Initial results suggested that NSE might indeed be a marker specific for neuroendocrine cells (48).
Sheppard et al. (46) studied the expression of NSE in pulmonary tumors and confirmed that this enzyme occurred exclusively in carcinoids and small cell carcinomas. Almost all carcinoids were positive whereas only 50% of the small cell carcinomas expressed this marker. Subsequent studies have shown that NSE can also be found in non-neuroendocrine cells. In a recent study on lung cancer (45), NSE immunoreactivity was demonstrated in all small cell carcinomas and carcinoids but also in about 50% of non-small cell carcinomas. A reason for this apparent

discrepancy may be that the available commercial anti-NSE antibodies have appeared to be insufficiently specific. Taken together, these findings suggest that NSE immunoreactivity may serve as a screening characteristic for the identification of neuroendocrine tumors but that the lack of specificity precludes its use for the definitive classification of pulmonary as well as other neuroendocrine neoplasms. A number of other enzymes, mostly involved in the metabolism of bioactive amines, has also been explored as marker for neuroendocrine differentiation. Histaminase and dopadecarboxylase have been advocated as markers for medullary carcinoma of the thyroid (29) but their use as markers for other neuroendocrine tumors has not been systematically studied. Furthermore, creatine kinase B/B has been studied in relation to small cell lung cancer (17). High levels of this enzyme were found in small cell carcinoma patients and also in tumor tissues. It is, however, probably not specific for lung carcinoma and therefore its diagnostic use, although as yet not systematically explored, may be limited.

A relatively new neuroendocrine marker is **chromogranin**, a protein which seems to occur in all neuroendocrine granules, regardless of their hormone content (30). The exclusive expression of chromogranin in a variety of neuroendocrine tumors, including pulmonary neoplasms, has been reported recently, indicating that this protein might indeed be highly specific for neuroendocrine differentiation. The presence of chromogranin was found to be strongly correlated with the results of Grimelius staining. Furthermore, the extent of its immunoreactivity appeared to be closely related to the density of neuroendocrine granules (45). Chromogranin may well be the most specific marker for neuroendocrine differentiation presently available. The absence of chromogranin immunoreactivity in tumors with only few neuroendocrine granules, however, limits its use as a marker for small cell lung cancer. The establishment of its reliability as a general neuroendocrine marker awaits further confirmation.

Epithelial cells have been shown to contain specific plasma membrane associated glycoproteins. Polyclonal as well as monoclonal antibodies have been generated against such antigens, using milk fat globule membranes as immunogen. The antigens recognized by these antibodies have been designated **epithelial membrane antigen** (EMA, 21) and **human milk fat globule related** antigen (HMFG, 49; MFGRA, 3). Considering the different patterns of immunoreactivity which are obtained with different antibodies, it is clear that they do not recognize the same antigen. Several studies on the immunolocalization of these antigens have been published. Most lung carcinomas express these antigens, regardless of the subtype (3, 31). Several investigators have attempted to use these antigens to distinguish between primary or metastatic pulmonary adenocarcinoma and mesothelioma. Marshall et al. (31), using two HMFG specific monoclonal antibodies, demonstrated expression of these antigens in most carcinomas as well as in most mesotheliomas. Benign mesothelium, however, did not express these antigens. Battifora & Kopinski (3) described a monoclonal antibody (MFG-2) which recognizes an antigen exclusively expressed by carcinoma cells and undetectable on neoplastic, reactive or normal mesothelium. This antibody therefore might be useful in the differentiation between adenocarcinoma (primary or metastatic) and mesothelioma.

Undoubtedly one of the most important developments in the immunodiagnosis of human neoplasms is the use of antibodies against **intermediate filament** proteins. The biochemical and cell biological characteristics of these proteins and their significance in tumor pathology have been reviewed extensively elsewhere (36, 40). Five classes of intermediate filament proteins can be distinguished: a) cytokeratins, a group of related proteins which almost exclusively occur in keratinizing and non keratinizing epithelia; b) vimentin, mainly restricted to mesenchymal cells; c) desmin, which occurs exclusively in smooth as well as striated muscle cells; d) neurofilament proteins, a group of at least 3 different

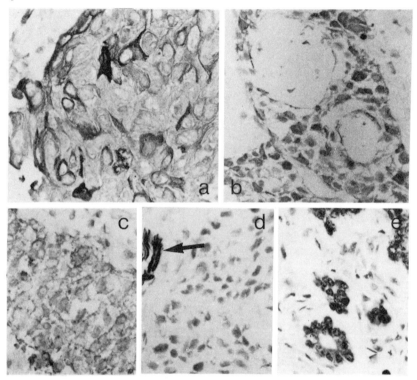

Fig. 5 Intermediate filament immunoreactivity in lung tumors. a. cytokeratin in squamous cell carcinoma; b. cytokeratin in adenocarcinoma; c. cytokeratin in SCC; d. neurofilament in SCC; tumor cells are negative, a nerve fiber (➡) is positively stained; e. cytokeratin in a carcinoid. (a-d frozen sections; e. paraffin sections; indirect immunoperoxidase, 250 x).

proteins which occur exclusively in neuronal cells and e) glial fibrillary acidic protein, which is found only in glial cells. Most cells therefore, under natural conditions, contain only one type of intermediate filament protein, a notable exception being muscle cells which contain desmin as well as vimentin. This pattern of intermediate filament protein expression is retained in neoplastic cells and therefore their immunocytochemical detection can be used for tumor classification. An interesting additional feature of the group of cytokeratins is that keratinizing and glandular epithelia show specific patterns of cytokeratin polypeptide expression, which are also retained in neoplastic cells (37).

Several groups have investigated patterns of intermediate filament expression in pulmonary neoplasms. All agree that in squamous cell carcinoma, adenocarcinoma, large cell carcinoma and mesothelioma cytokeratins occur (28, 34, 42, 44). Patterns of cytokeratin expression in pulmonary neoplasms are illustrated in fig. 5. With regard to small cell carcinomas, however, conflicting results have been reported. Lehto et al. (28) found only neurofilament expression in small cell carcinomas whereas Van Muyen et al. (34) detected only cytokeratin expression in these tumors. Similarly, Blobel et al., (5) found only cytokeratins in lung carcinoids and small cell carcinomas. The explanation for this discrepancy is not clear. Conceivably, the various monoclonal antibodies which were used in these studies may detect different epitopes. Furthermore it is possible that small cell carcinomas are a heterogeneous group of neoplasms. In this context the recent discovery of expression of neurofilament proteins in small cell carcinoma cell lines of variant subtype (11) is of interest.

3.4 Monoclonal antibody defined substances

The development of the hybridoma methodology for the production of monoclonal antibodies has provided an important tool for the recognition of antigens, exclusively or preferentially expressed by various human tumors. In recent years a wide variety of monoclonal antibodies has been generated against many different human tumors. Initially it was hoped that monoclonal antibodies could lead to the identification of tumor specific, organ specific or cell type specific antigens. Extensive characterisation of the majority of anti-tumor monoclonal antibodies, however, has shown that tumor specific antigens are rare, if they exist at all. The search for tissue or cell type specific antigen has been more succesful, although also in this area many initial claims of specificity appeared premature when the reactivity of the monoclonal antibody was tested on large numbers of various tumors and normal tissues. Nevertheless, monoclonal antibodies have demonstrated potential usefulness for various clinical applications, including immunohis-tochemical diagnosis and classification of primary cancers (16, 35).

Also for the study of lung cancer monoclonal antibodies have been developed. The available information on the antibodies that have been tested in immunohistochemical studies is listed in table II.

Brenner et al. (9) developed monoclonal antibodies reactive with squamous cell lung carcinomas. They did not test the reactivity on extrapulmonary squamous cells cancers. Most investigators have attempted to obtain monoclonal antibodies specific for small cell lung cancer.

The majority of these antibodies, however, when tested on various lung tumor cells lines, preferentially reacted with SCLC cell lines, although one of the antibodies described by Tong et al. (50) also reacted with non-SCLC cell lines. Some antibodies furthermore displayed strong reactivity with neuroblastoma cell lines (41). An important limitation of almost all of these studies is that the reactivity of the monoclonal antibodies was only tested on cancer cell lines. It is a general experience that testing on large panels of human cancer tissues often reveals more extensive reactivity patterns than was anticipated on the basis of test results on cancer cell lines. As yet, none of these antibodies have been applied for the histopathological diagnosis and classification of lung cancer. Consequently, their value as reagents for the differentiation between small-cell and non small-cell lung cancer remains to be established.

Table II. Characteristics of lung tumor reactive monoclonal antibodies.

Designation	Reactivity pattern	Corresponding antigen	Reference
9.2.2.	squamous cell cancer	30 kD protein	9
SM-1	SCLC (1)	25-50 kD protein	4
SCLC 2051	SCLC	25-30 kD protein	50
SCLC 2053	most types of lung cancer	u.n. (2)	50
600 series	SCLC, less on non-SCLC	glycolipids	41
SCCL 41,114, 124, 175	preferentially SCLC	u.n.	1

1) SCLC = small cell lung cancer
2) u.n. = unknown

4.   APPLICATIONS OF MARKER IMMUNOHISTOCHEMISTRY IN LUNG CANCER
     Immunocytochemical detection of markers can be of potential value 1) for the histopathological diagnosis and classification of primary lung cancers; 2) for the differentiation between primary and metastatic pulmonary neoplasms; 3) for the determination of the origin of metastatic pulmonary neoplasms and 4) as indicators of prognosis.

4.1 Histopathological diagnosis and classification of primary lung cancers
     Significant problems in this area are the differentiation between small-cell and non small-cell tumors, between large cell carcinoma and poorly differentiated squamous cell or adenocarcinoma and between adeno-carcinoma and mesothelioma. At present, the best markers for small-cell carcinoma (SCLC) appear to be the neuroendocrine markers neuron-specific

enolase, chromogranin and bombesin or GRP. Neuron-specific enolase reacts with most small-cell carcinomas but is not entirely specific. Chromogranin on the contrary appears to be highly specific but only reacts with SCLC with relative abundance of neuroendocrine granules. This probably holds true also for GRP. Therefore, concomitant application of these markers may be the best way to identify SCLC in cases of doubt. In addition, further testing of monoclonal SCLC reactive antibodies may result in additional reliable SCLC markers.

Although the clinical relevance of this problem is limited, the differentiation between large cell anaplastic carcinoma and poorly differentiated variants of squamous cell carcinoma or adenocarcinoma can be difficult. In this situation the use of monoclonal antibodies specific for subtypes of cytokeratin polypeptides may be of help. Immunoreactivity for cytokeratin polypeptides 18 and 19 is exclusively found in keratinizing epithelia and their presence in an anaplastic carcinoma is indicative of squamous differentiation. Similarly, immunoreactivity for cytokeratin polypeptides 5, 6 and 14-17 is exclusively found in glandular epithelia and their occurrence in an anaplastic carcinoma indicates adeno-differentiation (33) In this context, however, it should be kept in mind that in a significant proportion of lung carcinomas multiple lines of differentiation exist (32), which may complicate the use of marker expression patterns for tumor classification. Morphological criteria still remain the most important basis for lung tumor classification.

For the differentiation between adenocarcinoma and mesothelioma CEA seems to be the most reliable marker. In view of the fact that occasionally mesotheliomas exhibit CEA immunoreactivity, a combination of staining for CEA and for the MFG-2 defined antigens (3) which does not occur on mesotheliomas, may be more reliable.

4.2 Differentiation between primary and metastatic pulmonary neoplasms

Antigens exclusively expressed on bronchopulmonary epithelial cells and on their derivative tumors have not been found as yet. An exception appears to be the surfactant apoprotein, which is expressed only in bronchiolo- alveolar carcinomas with pneumocyte type II-like differentiation. Expression of this antigen by a lung adenocarcinoma clearly establishes its pulmonary origin.

4.3 Determination of the origin of metastatic pulmonary neoplasms

This problem will usually concern metastatic adenocarcinomas. The determination of their origin relies entirely on the availability of primary organ-specific antigens. A limited number of such antigens is available. Prostate specific acid phosphatase and prostate specific antigen are reliable markers of prostatic origin, thyroglobulin of thyroid origin and the OC 125 antigen (25) of ovarian origin. The histopathological diagnosis of metastatic disease is further discussed in chapter 11.

4.4 Indicators of prognosis

The availability of markers, of which the expression would predict the biological behaviour of a particular tumor type, clearly would be of major clinical significance. As yet, however, such markers have not been described. Conceivably, monoclonal antibody defined antigens may provide additional clues. For the moment correct histological classification, if necessary complemented with marker immunocyto-chemistry, remains the most solid basis for the prediction of the biological behaviour of pulmonary neoplasms.

REFERENCES

1. Ball ED, Graziano RF, Pettengill OS, Sorenson GD, Fanger MW (1984). Monoclonal antibodies reactives with small cell carcinomas of the lung. J. Natl. Cancer Inst. 72: 593-598.

2. Barsky SH, Rao NC, Restrepo C, Liotta LA (1984). Immunocytochemical enhancement of basement membrane antigens by pepsin: Applications in diagnostic pathology. Am.J.Clin.Pathol. 82: 191-194.

3. Battifora and Kopinski (1985). Distinction of mesothelioma from adenocarcinoma. An immunohistochemical approach. Cancer 55: 1679-1685).

4. Bernal SD, Speak JA (1984). Membrane antigens in small cell carcinoma of the lung defined by monoclonal antibody SM1. Cancer Res. 44: 265-270.

5. Blobel GA, Gould VE, Moll R, Lee I, Hseszar M, Geiger B, Franke W (1985). Coexpression of neuroendocrine markers and epithelial cytoskeletal proteins in bronchopulmonary neoplasms. Lab. Invest. 52: 39-51.

6. Bosman FT (1983). Some recent developments in immunocytochemistry. Histochem. J. 15: 189-200.

7. Bosman FT (1984). Neuroendocrine cells in non-neuroendocrine tumors. In: Evolution and Tumour Pathology of the Neuroendocrine system (Eds. S Falkmer, R Hakanson, F Sundler). Elsevier Sci Publ., p. 519-543.

8. Bosman FT, Brutel de la Riviere A, Giard RWM, Verhofstad AAJ, Cramer- Knijnenburg G (1984). Amine and peptide hormone production by lung carcinoid: a clinicopathological and immunocytochemical study. J. Clin.Pathol. 37: 931-936.

9. Brenner BG, Jothy S, Shuster J, Fuks A (1982). Monoclonal antibodies to human lung tumor antigens demonstrated by immunofluorescence and immunoprecipitation. Cancer Res. 42: 3187-3192.

10. Broder LE (1979). Hormone production by bronchogenic carcinoma: A review. Pathobiology Annual 9: 205-224.

11. Broers JLV, Rot MK, Wagenaar SjSc, Vooijs GP, Carney DN, Ramaekers FCS (1985). Intermediate filament expression in small cell lung cancer. In: Pathology and Biology of Lung Cancer (W. Bakker, ed.) University of Leiden, p. 110, abstract.

12. Carson JM, Pinkus GS (1982). Mesothelioma: Profile of keratin

proteins and carcinoembryonic antigen. An immunoperoxidase study of 20 cases and comparison with pulmonary adenocarcinomas. Am.J.Pathol. 108: 80-87.

13. Cutz E, Chan W, Track NS (1981). Bombesin, calcitonin and leu-enkephalin immunoreactivity in endocrine cells of human lung. Experienta 37: 765-766.

14. Dairaku M, Sueishi K, Tanaka K, Horie A (1983). Immunohistological analysis of surfactant-apoprotein in the bronchiolo-alveolar carcinoma. Virch.Arch. 400: 223-234.

15. Erlandson RA (1984). Diagnostic immunohistochemistry of human tumors. Am.J.Surg.Pathol. 8: 615-624.

16. Gatter KC, Mason DY (1982). The use of monoclonal antibodies for histopathological diagnosis of human malignancy. Semin.Oncol. 9: 517-525.

17. Gazdar AF, Zweig MH, Carney DN, Van Steirteghem AC, Baylin SB, Minna JD (1981). Levels of creatine kinase and its BB isoenzyme in lung cancer specimens and cultures. Cancer Res 41: 2773-2777.

18. Ghosh AK, Spriggs AI, Taylor-Papadimitriou J, Mason DY (1983). Immunocytochemical staining of cells in pleural and peritoneal effusions with a panel of monoclonal antibodies. J. Clin.Pathol. 36: 1154-1164.

19. Gould VE, Linnoila RI (1982). Pulmonary neuroepithelial bodies, neuroendocrine cells, and pulmonary tumors. Human Pathol. 13: 1064-1066.

20. Gould VE, Linnoila RI, Memoli VA, Warren WH (1983). Neuroendocrine cells and neuroendocrine neoplasms of the lung. Pathol. Ann. 18: 287-330.

21. Heyderman E, Steele K, Ormerod MG (1979). A new antigen on the epithelial membrane: its immunoperoxidase localization in normal and neoplastic tissue. J. Clin.Pathol. 32: 35-42.

22. Holden J, Churg A (1984). Immunohistochemical staining for keratin and carcinoembryonic antigen in the diagnosis of malignant mesothelioma. Am.J. Surg.Pathol. 8: 277-279.

23. Imura H (1980). Ectopic hormone syndromes. Clinics in Endocrinology and Metabolism 9: 235-260.

24. Kameya T, Shimosato Y, Kodama T, Tsumuraya M, Koide T, Yamaguchi K, Abe K (1983). Peptide hormone production by adenocarcinomas of the lung: Its morphologic basis and histogenetic considerations. Virch. Arch. 400: 245-257.

25. Kawabat SE, Bast RC Jr, Welch WR, Knapp RC, Colvin RB (1983). Immunopathologic characterization of a monoclonal antibody that

recognizes common surface antigens of human ovarian tumors of serous, endometrial and clear cell type. Am.J.Clin. Pathol. 79: 98-104.

26. Kloppel G, Girard J, Polak JM, Vaitukaitis JL, Kasper M, Heitz PU (1983). Alpha-human chorionic gonadotropin and neuron-specific enolase as markers for malignancy and neuroendocrine nature of pancreatic endocrine tumors. Cancer detection and prevention 6: 161-166.

27. Kwee WS, Veldhuizen RW, Golding RP, Mullink H, Stam J, Donner R, Boon ME (1982). Histologic distinction between malignant mesothelioma, benign pleural lesion and carcinoma metastasis. Evaluation of the application of morphometry combined with histochemistry and immunostaining. Virch.Arch. 397: 287-299.

28. Lehto VP, Stenman S, Miettinen M, Dahl D, Virtanen I (1983). Expression of a neural type of intermediate filament as a distinguishing feature between oat cell carcinoma and other lung cancers. Am. J. Pathol. 110: 113-118.

29. Lippman SM, Mendelsohn G, Trump DL, Wells SA, Baylin SB (1982). The prognostic and biological significance of cellular heterogeneity in medullary thyroid carcinoma: a study of calcitonin, L-Dopa decarboxylase and histaminase. J. Clin. Endocrinol. Metab. 54: 233-240.

30. Lloyd RV, Wilson B (1983). Specific endocrine tissue marker defined by a monoclonal antibody. Science 222: 628-630.

31. Marhsall RJ, Herbert A, Braye SG, Jones DB (1984). Use of antibodies to carcinoembryonic antigen and human milk fat globule to distinguish carcinoma, mesothelioma, and reactive mesothelium. J. Clin.Pathol. 37: 1215-1221.

32. McDowell EM, Trumpf BF (1983). Histogenesis of preneoplastic and neoplastic lesions in tracheobronchial epithelium. Surv.Synth. Pathol. Res. 2: 235- 279.

33. Moll RM, Franke W, Schiller DL, Geiger B, Krepler R (1982). The catalog of human cytokeratins patterns of expression in normal epithelium, tumors and cultured cells. Cell 31: 11-24.

34. Muyen GP van, Ruiter DJ, van Leeuwen C, Prins FA, Rietsema K, Warnaar SO (1984). Cytokeratin and neurofilament in lung carcinomas. Am.J. Pathol. 116: 363-369.

35. Neville AM, Forster CS, Moshakis V, Gove M (1982). Monoclonal antibodies and human tumor pathology. Human Pathol. 13: 1067-1081.

36. Osborn M, Weber K (1982). Intermediate filaments: Cell type specific markers in differentiation and pathology. Cell 31: 303-306.

37. Osborn M, Weber K (1983). Biology of disease. Tumor diagnosis by intermediate filament typing: A novel tool for surgical pathology. Lab. Invest. 48: 372-394.

38. Paladugu RR, Benfield JR, Pak HY, Ross RK, Teplitz RL (1985). Bronchopulmonary Kulchitsky cell carcinomas: a new classification scheme for typical and atypical carcinoids. Cancer 55: 1303-1311.

39. Pinkus GS, O'Connor EM, Etheridge CL, Corson JM (1985). Optimal immunoreactivity of keratin proteins in formalin fixed paraffin-embedded tissues requires preliminary trypsinization. J. Histochem.Cytochem. 33: 465-473.

40. Ramaekers FCS, Puts JJG, Moesker O, Kant A, Huysmans A, Haag D, Jap PHK, Herman CJ, Vooijs GP (1983). Antibodies to intermediate filament proteins in the immunohistochemical identification of human tumours: an overview. Histochem. J. 15: 691-713.

41. Rosen ST, Mulshine JL, Cuttitta F, Fedorko J, Carney DN, Gazdar A, Minna JD (1984). Analysis of human small cell lung cancer differentiation antigens using a panel of rat monoclonal antibodies. Cancer Res. 44: 2052-2061.

42. Saba SR, Espinoza CG, Richman AV, Azar HA (1983). Carcinomas of the lung: an ultrastructural and immunocytochemical study. Am.J. Clin.Pathol. 80: 6-13.

43. Said W, Nash G, Tepper G, Banks-Schlegel S (1983). Keratin proteins and carcinoembryonic anigen in lung carcinoma: An immunoperoxidase study of fifty-four cases, with ultrastructural correlations. Human Pathol. 14: 70-76.

44. Said W, Nash G, Banks-Schlegel S, Sassoon AF, Murakami S, Shintaku IP (1983b). Keratin in human lung tumors. Am.J.Pathol. 113: 27-32.

45. Said W, Vimadalal S, Nash G, Shintaku PI, Heusser RC, Sassoon AF, Lloyd RV (1985). Immunoreactive neuron-specific enolase, bombesin and chromogranin as markers for neuroendocrine lung tumors. Human Pathol. 16: 236-240.

46. Sheppard MN, Conin B, Bennett MH (1984). Immunocytochemical localization of neuron-specific enolase in small cell carcinoma and carcinoid tumors of the lung. Histopathol. 8: 171-182.

47. Sidhu GS (1979). The endodermal origin of digestive and respiratory tract APUD-cells. Am.J.Pathology 96: 5-20.

48. Tapia FJ, Polak JM, Barbosa AJA (1981). Neuron-specific enolase is produced by neuroendocrine tumors. Lancet 1: 808-811.

49. Taylor-Papadimitriou J, Peterson JA, Arklie J, Burchell J, Ceriani RI, Bodmer WF (1981). Monoclonal antibodies to epithelium-specific components of human milk fat globule membrane: production and reaction with cells in culture. Int.J. Cancer 28: 17-21.

50. Tong AW, Lee J, Stone MJ (1984). Characterization of two human small cell lung carcinoma-reactive monoclonal antibodies generated by a novel immunization approach. Cancer Res. 44: 4987-4992.

51. Wachner R, Wittekind C, von Kleist S (1984). Localisation of CEA, -HCG, SP1, and keratin in the tissue of lung carcinomas. A histochemical study. Virch.Arch. 402: 415-423.

52. Wang N, Huang S, Gold P (1979). Absence of carcinoembryonic antigen-like material in mesothelioma. An immunohistochemical differentiation from other lung cancers. Cancer 44: 937-943.

53. Warren WH, Memoli VA, Gould VE (1984). Immunohistochemical and ultrastructural analysis of bronchopulmonary neuroendocrine neoplasms. I. Carcinoids. Ultrastructural Pathology 6: 15-27.

54. Whitaker D, Shilkin KB (1981). Carcinoembryonic antigen in tissue diagnosis of malignant mesothelioma. Lancet 1981/i: 1369.

55. Yang K, Ulich Th, Taylor I, Cheng L, Lewin KJ (1983). Pulmonary carcinoids. Immunohistochemical demonstration of brain-gut peptides. Cancer 52: 819-823.

CRITICAL EVALUATION OF NEW TECHNIQUES IN THE MORPHOLOGICAL DIAGNOSIS OF LUNG CANCER

J.D. ELEMA , L. DE LEIJ , P. POSTMUS , S. POPPEMA , T.H. THE

1. INTRODUCTION

The group of lungancers constitutes the most important cause of cancer-ueath in men and its incidence rapidly increases in women (1). According to the WHO classification (2) the main types are Squamous Cell Cancer (SCC), Small Cell Lung Cancer (SCLC), Adenocarcinoma (AC) and Large Cell Anaplastic Cancer (LCC), together embracing about 95% of all lungtumors.
This classification is based on light-microscopic criteria.

The introduction of fibreoptic bronchoscopy in the diagnosis of lung-cancer has considerably added to the difficulties encountered by the pathologist in arriving at a diagnosis as demonstrated by Chuang e.a. (3). This biopsy technique yields tiny pieces of tissue from which conclusions with far-reaching consequences have to be drawn. Are "new techniques" of any help in this dilemma? As demonstrated by a study of Feinstein e.a. (4) there is considerable variability in judgement among different pathologists and even individual pathologists may vary in their diagnosis. Not surprisingly variation especially concerns poorly differentiated tumors. The question therefore arises whether the use of "new techniques" may help in improving the consistency in diagnosis and in better defining difficult and poorly differentiated tumors. Finally as a third area of daily sores we will consider the problem of the diagnosis of proliferative pleural lesions and especially the question whether the use of "new techniques" is of any help in differentiating between malignant mesothelioma and pleural invasion of adenocarcinoma.

What should be included in the heading of "new techniques"? Obviously this paper is primarily concerned with the daily practice of lungcancer diagnosis and we will therefore restrict ourselves to histological techniques other than conventional paraffin embedding and standard histochemical staining as far as they are daily practice in major centres at this moment. Techniques to be discussed are the possibilities of plastic embedding, electron-microscopy and immunohistochemistry. To what extent and in which way can these techniques be applied in smaller pathology departments?

2. THE PROBLEM OF SMALL (BRONCHIAL) BIOPSIES

Although problems encountered in dealing with small fibreoptic biopsies have been illustrated for non-SCLC (3) considerable uncertainty may also exist when a decision has to be made on the possible presence of SCLC.

In fact, given the present state of treatment the single most important
decision is that of SCLC versus non-SCLC. But also every effort of course
should be made to arrive at a specific diagnosis in cases of non-SCLC.
Plastic embedding. For a number of years we have routinely embedded
formalin fixed bronchial biopsies in glycolmethacrylate (5) followed by
cutting with glass knives and conventional H&E staining of 2 µ sections.
Dehydration of the tissue and impregnation with glycolmethacrylate takes
place in a Histokinette system overnight. Embedding with polymerization is
done during the following morning so that sections will be ready in the
afternoon. The procedure generally takes a few more hours than the paraffin
procedure. Polymerization is crucial and can be speeded by incubation at a
temperature of 40°-60°C. As so often, the best approach has to be selected
by varying the directions given by the manufacturers. We have made use
of chemicals and instructions of both Du Pont company (Sorvall)* and
Kulzer & Co (Histoset)* with good results. Plastic sections are undoubtedly of more stable and better quality than paraffin (paraplast) sections in
our hands. There is no shrinkage of any importance and morphological and
cytological details are well preserved. This difference in quality is nice-
ly demonstrated in figures 1 and 2. Figure 1 is from an H&E stained
paraffin section of a bronchial biopsy labeled as a possible SCLC. The
tissue was transferred from the paraffin to plastic and figure 2 is from an
H&E stained plastic section cut at the same thickness. The eventual diagnosis was poorly differentiated SCC.

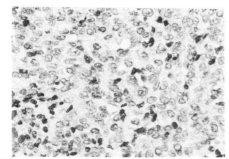 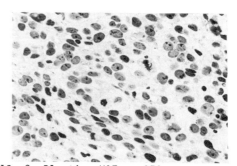

FIG. 1. Paraffin, H&E, x 350   FIG. 2. Plastic, H&E, x 350

An important disadvantage of the plastic embedding is that immunehistochemistry is not easily performed in a routine way. So if one wants to
keep the option of performing immunehistochemistry on a routine basis (see
later) tissue should be embedded in paraffin or, preferably, two biopsies
should be taken. One of these can be used for plastic embedding, the other
can be quick frozen to be used for immunehistochemistry. Clearly the
"paraffin-only" approach is not ideal.
Electron-microscopy. The application of electron microscopy for the study
of lungtumors has resulted in fundamental changes of concepts on the histogenesis of lungcancer (6, 7, 8, 9). Ultrastructural studies have revealed
details, not visible with the light-microscope, that can be used in
classification especially in cases of poorly- or undifferentiated cancers.
In this way it was shown that LCC's often represent either poorly differentiated AC's or poorly differentiated SCC's (10). Occasionally a

---

* Du Pont company, Newton, Conn. U.S.A.
**Kulzer & Co. GmbH, D-6393, Wehrheim/Ts, BRD.

diagnosis of LCC was changed into that of a "neuroendocrine" tumor (11). Both Saba e.a. (11) and Auerbach e.a. (12) also show that in fact adeno-squamous cancers are, judged by electron-microscopy, the most frequent category of lung cancer. Whether such findings, given the problems of sampling error, should lead to a change of diagnosis is a matter to be discussed later. At any rate, using electron-microscopic criteria, the light-microscopic diagnosis was changed or classified more precisely in 20 of 52 and 26 of 49 cases respectively in the aforementioned publications. These results show the possible usefulness of applying electron-microscopy in bronchial biopsies. These biopsies themselves have the inherent and accepted disadvantage of sampling error. As they can be processed in toto electron-microscopy does not further add to this problem. We have studied 226 consecutive bronchial biopsies with electron-microscopy using established criteria for the different types of cancer (6, 11, 13). To this purpose biopsies were immediately put into glutaraldehyde 2% and embedded in Epon. A light-microscopic diagnosis was made on 2 sections stained according to Flores and Hoffman (14). A total of 96 biopsies contained infiltrative cancer, 5 cases were suspected for cancer and 2 cases were equivocal. In the 5 biopsies suspected for cancer this could be ruled out in one case. Suspicion of SCLC in three biopsies with cancer was confirmed. A change of diagnosis took place in 13 instances and in 4 of these this concerned a change into SCLC (Table 1).

TABLE 1.   EM in bronchial biopsies

LM	?	Susp.	Susp.SCLC	SCLC	SCC	ACC	LCC	Carcin.
?	2/2							
Suspect		4/5						
Susp. SCLC			0/3	3/3				
SCLC				38/38				
SCC				2/40	36/40	2/40		
AC					1/4	3/4		
LCC				2/10	5/10	1/10	2/10	
Carcinoid								1/1
EM/LM:	2/2	4/5	0/3	45/38	42/40	6/4	2/10	1/1

(Number of LM diagnoses is given in denominator, of EM in nominator).

The largest single light-microscopic group that was reclassified was the group of LCC. In two instances this diagnosis was changed into SCLC (fig. 3 and 4).
    Four SCC's and one AC were also changed. In going back over the light-microscopic slides we concluded that in fact the diagnosis in these cases and in a number of others as well had been made on the general appearance rather than on strict criteria. Our results show that the use of electron-microscopy may considerably influence the histological diagnosis of lung-cancer. However, given the high cost and the time-consuming procedure it is not a tool for routine application. Although work-up of the material can be done within a day, as was the case in our study, this would mean special and preferential treatment for all bronchial biopsies taken for possible cancer bringing along a considerable burden with the risk of jeopardizing other activities. The main problem of course in using electron-microscopy

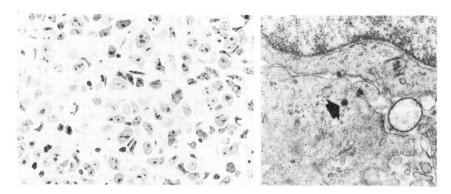

FIG. 3. Undifferentiated cancer labeled as LCC. Note presence of nucleoli.
(x 350). FIG. 4. EM of same biopsy. Several typical dense-core granules
were found in the absence of features indicating either SCC or AC.
Granule indicated by arrow.

for routine diagnosis is the fact that it is generally not available outside the larger (academic) centres. It is our feeling that electron-microscopy of bronchial biopsies taken for the diagnosis of lung cancer is not
competitive because of high cost and limited availability. It is however
a very sensitive tool.
Immunohistochemistry. This technique has the advantage that by now it is
available in most pathology departments, and if not it should be so. It is
much cheaper than electron-microscopy and also much quicker. An important
problem with small biopsies is the amount of tissue available and how to
use it. Quality control both of the antisera used and of the histological
technique is imperative as again stressed by Dranoff and Birgner (15).
Table 2 lists a number of antisera that might be considered useful in
differentiating SCLC from non-SCLC. Only antisera are listed that are
commercially and therefore generally available.

TABLE 2.

			Immunehistochemistry of SCLC		
			SCLC	Carcinoid	non-SCLC
Neurofil.	ref. 23	P,F	+		-
	ref. 24	F	0/9		1/16
	*	F	1/9		-
NSE	ref. 20	P	1/2		-
	ref. 18	P	3/3		
	ref. 19	?	5/5		
	ref. 21	P	18/31	16/18	-
MOC-1	*	F	9/9	1/1	-**
S100	*	P	0/4		-
ACTH	ref. 16	P	3/22	14/22	
Bombesin	ref. 16	P	6/22	3/22	
Leu-7		P	Reported to be + in some SCLC		
(HNK-1	ref. 26)				

*Own experience. Monoclonal antibodies directed against Neurofilament (kd
210) and "MOC-1" were obtained from Eurodiagnostics, BV, Apeldoorn, the
Netherlands, anti S100 was obtained from DAKO. P indicates paraffin, F
frozen sections. **Focal weak staining in some cases.

Most of these antisera can be used on paraffin sections. The low frequency of positive results for staining of hormones (16) argues against its routine use. S-100 protein is associated with neuroectodermal tissue and its tumors (17). We obtained negative results in SCLC. The use of Neuron-Specific Enolase (NSE) for the detection of SCLC has been reported by several groups. Either all cases tested (18, 19) or a considerable number of them (20, 21) stained positive. Some warning should be expressed. Vinores et al.(20) have shown that NSE may be present in tumors not related to the nervous system or to the APUD-system. It has not been found in non-neuro-endocrine lungcancers so far. Our own experience is limited and not very satisfactory. It may be that fixation is very crucial as implied by Jaffe and Yunis (22) and by the variable results of the authors mentioned. The presence of neurofilaments in SCLC has been used by Lehto (23) as a reliable diagnostic criterium. This has not been confirmed for reasons not yet known (24). We have now considerable experience with our monoclonal "MOC-1" reacting in a homogenous and strong manner with all our cases of SCLC (fig. 5) except for one cytological preparation (25).

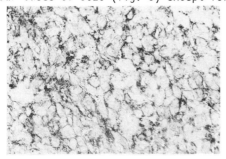

This antibody is not completely specific, some focal weak staining has been detected in a few other cancers that are currently being reviewed. A disadvantage as with many monoclonal antibodies is the fact that it can only be used on frozen material. HNK-1 was demonstrated in paraffin sections of neuro-endocrine tumors (26) and may be useful for detection of SCLC. Our own experience is very limited and not satisfying. We conclude from the literature that staining for NSE in paraffin sections may be used with some caveats. We prefer to use

FIG. 5. MOC-1 staining of SCLC
      (x 350).

MOC-1 staining of frozen sections. Our advi e is to obtain two biopsies, one for light-microscopy for plastic embedding and one to be quick frozen for immunohistochemistry according to needs arising.

3. DIFFICULT AND POORLY DIFFERENTIATED TUMORS
    Even when apparently sufficient tissue is available it may be difficult to decide for instance whether an adenocarcinoma represents a primary lung-cancer or a metastasis. The heterogeneity of lungcancers has been established both by electron-microscopy (7, 10, 13, 27) and by light-microscopy (28). This adds to the problem of deciding on the basic character of poorly differentiated cancers. The question is therefore whether new techniques can help in solving such problems.
Histochemistry. When confronted with an adenocarcinomatous lesion of possible metastatic origin a positive staining for acetylsialomucin (29) may indicate the colon as the primary site of the tumor. The presence of PTAH-positive granules in tumor cells identifies a primary adenocarcinoma of the lung (30). We have no personal experience with the application of these procedures for these purposes.
Electron-microscopy. The great value of electron-microscopy in characterizing tumors of the lung has been mentioned earlier. Clara cells have been shown to be a frequent cell of origin of peripheral adenocarcinoma and bronchiolo-alveolar carcinoma (30, 31). The recognition of these cells and

alveolar type II cells in adenocarcinoma in lung or regional lymph nodes definitely rules out the possibility of metastatic tumor from a localization outside the lung. Fig. 6 demonstrates Clara cells in a left-sided supra-clavicular metastasis. On this basis a definite diagnosis of primary adenocarcinoma of the lung could be made in this patient. Thus application of electron-microscopy can be very rewarding in the area of lungtumors. Drawbacks have been mentioned before. Given the heterogeneity of lungtumors the problem of sampling error should be especially mentioned.

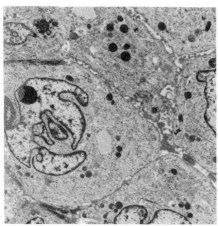

Immuno-histochemistry. In recent years a large number of studies have been published on the use of immunohisto-chemical methods for the analysis of tumors in general and also specifically of lungtumors. Emphasis has been on the detection of Carcino-Embryonic Antigen (CEA) and the intermediate filaments among which the keratins are the most interesting for lungtumors. The possible value of neurofilaments, S-100, NSE and MOC-1 has been commented on before. It should be mentioned that there is a preliminary report showing the presence of NSE and neurofilaments in a majority of Giant Cell Cancers (32). In discussing other possible markers we will restrict ourselves to CEA, Epithelial Membrane Antigen (EMA) and intermediate filaments to which antisera are commercially available.

FIG. 6. Clara-cells in metastatic lymph node. The electron-dense inclusions often contain finger-print-like lamellar structures.

Although mesenchymal tumors, especially malignant ones, are rare in the lung, diagnostic difficulties may arise because of the occasional sarcomatous growth pattern of squamous cancer. In these cases a search for the presence of the different intermediate filaments can be very helpful (33, 34, 35, 36, 37). In all articles dealing with the use of intermediate filaments as marker it has been stated that under "in vivo" circumstances tumors run true to their celltype of origin as far as the presence of their filaments is concerned. Mesenchymal tumors are characterized by vimentin, epithelial tumors by keratin. The demonstration of keratin or other epithelial antigens like CEA or EMA in apparently sarcomatous tumors indicates the epithelial, pseudosarcomatous character. Figure 7 demonstrates the value of this in a case in which it was difficult to decide between a carcinosarcoma and a pseudo-sarcomatous SCC. The presence of keratin in fusiform cells indicated the epithelial character. In using these polyclonal antibodies against intermediary filaments on paraffin embedded tissue it should be realized that these filaments are vulnerable and fixation and paraffin embedding may damage or mask the antigens (36), resulting in variable staining. As the array of commercially available antibodies to intermediary filaments will rapidly increase it is of the utmost importance that careful attention is given to the properties of these antibodies and the molecular weight of the filament against which they are directed. Proper controls should always be run. In view of the above mentioned uncertainties negative staining of paraffin sections for keratin does not rule out carcinoma. CEA and EMA are other antigens that may be used. Both are

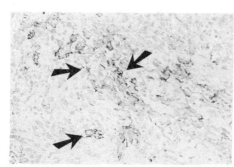

FIG. 7. Pseudosarcomatous SCC stained
for keratin (Paraffin, x 140).

well preserved in formalin-fixed,
paraffin embedded tissue and regular-
ly present in epithelial tumors of
the lung (38, 39, 40). The results
of CEA staining have been variable
judging from the literature.
Thorough absorption of some commercially available antisera is of
paramount importance as demonstrated
by Nap (40). Our further experience
with EMA staining of lungtumors
generally shows the same results as
those obtained for CEA.Neither of
these markers is useful for subtyping
of epithelial tumors (38).

Keratin immunohistochemistry. Nineteen different keratins have been recognized (41); the subject was recently reviewed by Cooper   (42). Keratins
can be divided in two subfamilies. Specific keratins from each subfamily
pair with each other and the expression of such pairs is related to type
of epithelium, differentiation programm and state of cellular growth.
According to Cooper   (42) practically all SCC's express 50-58, 48-56
and 46 kd keratins whereas neoplasms of simple epithelia express the smaller keratins. A large number of studies on keratins have been published (24,
32, 33, 36, 39, 43, 44, 45, 46, 47, 48) mostly using polyclonal antibodies
on paraffin-embedded material and without further specification of the
keratin-type. These antisera generally stain all SCC's, a variable proportion of AC's and LCC's and a minority of SCLC's. The single use of these
antisera appears not very fruitful except for demonstrating the epithelial
character of these tumors. The production of monoclonal antibodies against
specific keratins is more promising. Ramaekers(46) produced two
such antibodies one of which is directed against 45kd keratin. The other is
not specified but only reacts with keratinized material and therefore does
not give additional information. Presumably this antibody is directed
against one of the high MWt keratins. The antibody against the 45kd keratin
does not stain SCC which is in agreement with the experience and hypothesis
of Cooper   (42). Our own experience so far with this antibody is
limited and in agreement with that of Ramaeker: SCC's were negative, all
SCLC's and AC's were positive. Published data and our own experience mainly
concern well differentiated, recognizable tumors. Especially the poorly
differentiated tumors that are often classified differently by different
pathologists are an interesting group to further analyse with this and
other monoclonal antibodies that may become available. It is possible that
the presence or absence of the 45kd keratin in a tumor can be used as an
important discriminant in poorly differentiated tumors. It is our opinion
that in doing so one should rely on the use of monoclonal antibodies on
frozen sections. The results of Said   (47) for instance with polyclonal
monospecific antibodies on paraffin sections are not in agreement with
those of Cooper   (42) and Ramaekers   (46). When more of these
monoclonal antibodies become commercially available "keratin-fingerprinting"
of tumors becomes feasable as a routine tool. The reader is especially
referred to the article by Cooper   (42) for further reading on this
subject.

3. DIAGNOSIS OF MALIGNANT MESOTHELIOMA, DIFFERENTIATION FROM PLEURAL
   INFILTRATION OF ADENOCARCINOMA
   Pleural biopsies with atypical proliferations pose a frequent diagnostic
problem. Histochemical staining for hyaluronic acid is a first approach but
negative staining for Alcian Blue does not rule out malignant mesothelioma.
Recently several studies have been published that deal with the application
of immunohistochemistry to the problem. The most complete contributions are
those of Kwee (49) and more recently of Whitaker and Shilkin (50). In both
very useful studies it is stated that malignant mesotheliomas are negative
for CEA. Positive staining for CEA rules out malignant mesothelioma. As not
all cancers are CEA positive this test is not foolproof . Reports of
occasional positive staining of mesotheliomas (43, 47, 51) may have been
due to inadequate absorption of CEA-antisera. In our own limited experience
malignant mesotheliomas have always been negative. As reactive mesothelial
cells are also negative for CEA this procedure is of no help in differentiating between reactive and malignant mesothelial proliferations. Two
approaches have been taken to solve this problem. Kwee   (52) used
morphometry and concluded that the mean nuclear area of reactive mesothelial
cells is significantly smaller than that of malignant mesothelial cells.
There are no differences between mesotheliomas and carcinomas. To et al (53)
found immunohistochemical staining for EMA of pleural effusions valuable.
Strong positive staining of cells indicated malignancy. Depending on the
technique used considerable numbers of "false-negative" results may be
obtained. Whitaker and Shilkin (50) found reactive mesothelial cells negative or weakly staining whereas all malignant proliferations stained
strongly positive. We have no personal experience with either approach.
As a routine we use paraffin embedding of pleural biopsies suspected for
malignancies and staining for HE, hyaluronic acid (Alcian Blue without
and with hyaluronidase pretreatment), CEA and EMA. In view of the possible
social consequences of a diagnosis of mesothelioma it may be necessary to
revert to the use of EM. Both biopsies and pleural effusions can be used.
Electron-microscopy can be used to establish the mesothelial character of
the proliferating cells but not to decide whether this proliferation is
reactive or malignant.

5. IMPACT OF NEW TECHNIQUES ON DIAGNOSIS AND CLASSIFICATIONS OF LUNGTUMORS.
   Classification and daily practice of lungcancer diagnosis solely rests
on light-microscopic interpretation of tumor tissue most often embedded in
paraffin. Existing intra- and interobserver variability (4) may be caused
by poor preparation of the tissue and by a lack of clear-cut morphological
criteria or the careless application of these. A third important factor
may be the heterogenous nature of many lungcancers. Should the existing
classification therefore eventually be replaced by a new one and diagnosis
be based on the use of for instance immunohistochemistry and keratin
"finger-printing"? Both Sobin (54) and Nash (55) have addressed this question and conclude that light-microscopy also in the future should remain
the basis for classification and the first approach for making a diagnosis.
If additional morphological techniques are used,   their results should
be given in a qualified way in addition to the light-microscopic diagnosis.
In this way it will remain possible to compare data from centres all over
the world. It could be suggested that this statement is illusionary
because of existing observer variability. It is quite possible that this
variability can be reduced emphasizing the obligation of pathologists and
clinicians to strive for optimal handling and preparation of the tissue and
to refrain from casual application of diagnostic terms. The use of

Electron-microscopy and immunohistochemistry would be especially indicated in poorly- and undifferentiated tumors (55), but it is very likely that especially the use of immunohistochemistry in well characterized tumors will also give additional important data. Sappino (56) for instance suggested that the presence of "keratin" in SCLC might be of prognostic value. The impact therefore of new techniques recently available and to be developed is one of further tuning of classification and refinement of diagnosis. Light-microscopy will also in the future remain the backbone of tumor diagnosis. Everybody involved in handling and processing tissue for diagnosis has the obligation of doing this in an optimal way. Finally it should be remembered that a good working relation between clinician and pathologist can never be replaced by any sort of "new technique".

REFERENCES

1. Stolley D.
   Lung cancer in women - five years later, situation worse.
   New Engl.J.Med.1983,309:428.
2. The World Health Organization histological typing of lung tumors.
   World Health Organization.
   Am.J.Clin.Pathol.1982,12:123.
3. Chuang M.T. et al.
   Diagnosis of lung cancer by fibreoptic bronchoscopy: problems in the histological classification of non-small cell carcinomas.
4. Feinstein A.R., et al.
   Observer variability in the histopathologic diagnosis of lung cancer.
   Am.Rev.Resp.Dis.1970,101:671.
5. Bennett H.S. et al.
   Science and art in preparing tissues embedded in plastic for light-microscopy, with special reference to glycol metacrylate, glass knives and simple stains.
   Stain Technology 1976, 51:71.
6. Mc Dowell E.M. et al.
   The respiratory epithelium. V.Histogenesis of lung carcinoma in the human.
   J.Natl.Cancer Inst.1978,61:587.
7. Mc Dowell E.M. et al.
   Pulmonary endocrine tumors with mixed phenotypes - a hypothesis to explain their existence.
   Lab.Invest.1980, 42:134.
8. Tischler A.S.
   Small cell carcinoma of the lung: cellular origin and relationship to other neoplasms.
   Semin.Oncol.1978,5:244.
9. Yesner R.
   Spectrum of lung cancer and ectopic hormones.
   Pathol.Ann.1978,13(1): 217.
10. Churg A.
    The fine structure of large cell undifferentiated carcinoma of the lung: evidence for its relation to squamous cell carcinomas and adenocarcinomas.
    Human Pathol. 1978, 9:143.
11. Saba S.R. et al.
    Carcinomas of the lung: an ultrastructural and immunocytochemical study.
    Am.J.Clin.Pathol.1983,80:6.

12. Auerbach O.et al.
    A comparison of World Health Organization (WHO) classification of
    lung tumors by light and electron microscopy.
    Cancer 1982, 50:2079.
13. Sidhu G.
    The ultrastructure of malignant epithelial neoplasms of the lung.
    Pathol.Ann.1982,1:235.
14. Flores T.R., E.O.Hoffmann
    A rapid polychromatic staining method for semi-thin epon sections.
    Proc.Royal Microsc.Soc.1981,16:163.
15. Dranoff G., D.D.Bigner
    A word of caution in the use of neuron-specific enolase expression
    in tumor diagnosis.
    Arhc.Pathol.Lab.Med.1984,108:535.
16. Gould V.E. et al.
    Neuroendocrine cells and neuroendocrine neoplasma of the lung.
    Pathol.Ann.1983,1:287.
17. Kahn H.J. et al.
    Role of antibody to S100 protein in diagnostic pathology.
    Am.J.Clin.Pathol.1983,79:341.
18. Wick M.R. et al.
    Neuron-specific enolase in neuroendocrine tumors of the thymus,
    bronchus, and skin.
    Am.J.Clin.Pathol.1983,29:703.
19. Banner B.F. et al.
    Immunohistochemical demonstration of neuroendocrine markers in cyto-
    logic specimens.
    Lab.Invest.1985,52:5A.
20. Vinores S.A. et al.
    Immunohistochemical demonstration of neuron-specific enolase in neo-
    plasms of the CNS and other tissues.
    Arch.Pathol.Lab.Med.1984,108:536.
21. Sheppard M.N. et al.
    Immunocytochemical localization of neuron-specific enolase in small
    cell carcinomas and carcinoid tumours of the lung.
    Histopathology 1984, 8:171.
22. Jaffe R., E.J.Yunis
    Neuron-specific enolase is useful in the differential diagnosis of
    childhood round cell tumors.
    Lab.Invest.1983,48:7P.
23. Lehto V.P.et al.
    Expression of a neural type of intermediate filament as a distin-
    guishing feature between oat cell carcinoma and other lung cancers.
    Am.J.Pathol.1983,110:113.
24. Van Muyen G.N.P. et al.
    Cytokeratin and neurofilament in lung carcinomas.
    Am.J.Pathol.1984,116:363.
25. De Leij L. et al.
    The diagnostic use of monoclonal antibodies against small cell lung
    carcinoma cells.
    Neth.J.Med.1985,28:119.
26. Cailland J.M. et al.
    HNK-1 defined antigen detected in paraffin-embedded neuroectoderm
    tumors and those derived from cells of the amine precursor uptake
    and decarboxylation system.
    Cancer Res.1984,44:4432.

27. Mc Dowell E.M. et al.
    Pulmonary small cell carcinoma showing tripartitic differentiation in
    individual cells.
    Human Pathol. 1981, 12:286
28. Hirsch F.R.et al.
    Tumor heterogeneity in lung cancer based on light microscopic features.
    A retrospective study of a consecutive series of 2000 patients treated
    surgically.
    Virch.Arch. A 1983, 402:147.
29. Cooper J.H. and R.G.Durning
    An improved histochemical method for distinguishing colonic acetylsia
    lomucin from other epithelial mucins.
    J.Histochem. Cytochem. 1981, 29:1445.
30. Ogata T and K.Ando.
    Clara cell granules of peripheral lung cancers
    Cancer 1984, 54:1635.
31. Espinoza C.G. et al.
    Ultrastructural and immunohistochemical studies of bronchiolo-alveolas
    carcinomas.
    Cancer 1984, 54:2182.
32. Carlson G.J. et al.
    Coexpression of intermediate filaments in giant cell carcinoma of the
    lung.
    Lab.Invest.1985, 12:12A.
33. Ramaekers F.C.S et al.
    Differential diagnosis of human carcinomas, sarcomas and their meta-
    stases using antibodies to intermediate-sized filament.
    Eur.J. Cancer Clin.Oncol. 1982, 18:1251.
34. Denk H.et al.
    Proteins of intermediate filaments. An immunohistochemical and bio-
    chemical approach to the classification of soft tissue tumors.
    Am.J.Pathol. 1983, 110:193.
35. Osborn M.and K.Weber
    Biology of disease. Tumor diagnosis by intermediate filament typing:
    a novel tool for surgical pathology.
    Lab.Invest. 1983, 48:372.
36. Ramaekers F.C.S. et al.
    Antibodies to intermediate filament proteins in the immunohistochemical
    identifcation of human tumours: an overview.
    Histochemical Journal 1983, 15:691.
37. Damjanov I.
    Antibodies to intermediate filament and tumor diagnosis.
    Ultrastruct.Pathol. 1983, 4:1.
38. Sloane J.P. et al.
    Distribution of epithelial membrane antigen in normal and neoplastic
    tissues and its value in diagnostic tumor pathology.
    Cancer 1981, 47: 1786.
39. Said J.W. et al.
    Keratin proteins and carcinoembryonic antigen in lung carcinoma.
    An immunoperoxidase study of fifty-four cases, with ultrastructural
    correlations.
    Human Pathol. 1983, 14:70.
40. Nap M.
    Carcinoembryonic antigen. An immunohistologic study.
    Acad.Thesis, Groningen 1984.

102

41. Moll R. et al.
The catalog of human cytokeratins: pattern of expression in normal
epithelia, tumors and cultured cells.
Cell 1982, 31:11.
42. Cooper D. et al.
Classification of human epithelia and their neoplasms using monoclonal
antibodies to keratins: strategies, apllications and limitations.
Lab.Invest. 1985, 52:243.
43. Corson J.M. and G.S.Pinkus
Mesothelioma: a profile of keratin proteins and carcinoembryonic anti-
gen. An immunoperoxidase study of 20 cases and comparison with pulmo-
nary adenocarcinomas.
Am.J.Pathol. 1982, 108:80.
44. Gusterson G.et al.
Immunohistochemical localization of keratin in human lung tumors.
Virch.Arch.A 1982, 394:269.
45. Bejui-Thivolet F. et al.
Intracellular keratins in normal and pathological bronchial mucosa.
Immunocytochemical studies on biopsies and cell suspensions.
Virch.Arch. A 1982, 395:87.
46. Ramaekers F.C.S. et al.
Monoclonal antibody to keratin filaments, specific for glandular
epithelia and their tumors. Use in surgical pathology.
Lab.Invest. 1983, 49:353.
47. Said J.W. et al.
Keratin in human lung tumors. Patterns of localization of different-
molecular-weight keratin proteins.
Am.J.Pathol. 1983, 113:27.
48. Blobel G.A. et al.
Coexpression of neuroendocrine markers and epithelial cytoskeletal
proteins in bronchopulmonary neuroendocrine neoplasms.
Lab.Invest. 1985, 52:39.
49. Kwee W.S.
Quantitative and qualitative studies of malignant mesothelioma.
Acad.Thesis. Free University, Amsterdam, 1982.
50. Whitake D. and K.B.Shilkin
Diagnosis of pleural malignant mesothelioma in life. A practical
approach.
J.Pathol. 1984, 143:147.
51. Loosli H. and J.Hurlimann.
Immunohistological study of malignant diffuse mesotheliomas of the
pleura.
Histopathology 1984, 8:793.
52. Kwee W.S. et al
Histologic distinction between malignant mesothelioma, benign pleural
lesion and carcinoma metastasis. Evaluation of the application of
morphometry combined with histochemistry and immunostaining.
Virch Arch. A 1982, 397:287.
53. To A.et al.
Epithelial membrane antigen. Its use in the cytodiagnosis of malignancy
in serous effusions.
Am. J.Clin.Pathol. 1982, 78:214.
54. Sobin L.H.
The histologic classification of lung tumors: the need for a double
standard.
Human Pathol. 1983, 14:1020.

55. Nash G.
    The diagnosis of lung cancer in the 80's: will routine light micros-
    copy suffice?
    Human Pathol. 1983, 14:1021
56. Sappino A.P. et al.
    Immunohistochemical localisation of keratin in small cell carcinoma of
    the lung: correlation with response to combination chemotherapy.
    Eur. J.Cancer Clin. Oncol. 1983, 19:1365.

FLOW CYTOMETRIC DNA ANALYSIS IN THE STUDY OF SMALL CELL CARCINOMA OF THE LUNG

L.L. VINDELØV, S.Aa.ENGELHOLM and M.SPANG-THOMSEN

1. INTRODUCTION

An important aspect to consider in the design of combination chemotherapy for small cell carcinoma of the lung (SCCL), as well as for other types of malignancy, is tumor heterogeneity. Different subpopulations in a tumor may vary in cell kinetic behaviour and in sensitivity to various antineoplastic treatment. The ultimate outcome of the treatment seems to depend on how well the individual drugs in a combination, and the schedule in which they are given, match the sensitivity and cell kinetics of the subpopulations of each individual tumor.

Flow cytometric DNA analysis is rapid and accurate (7-11). It yields information of Gl-cell DNA content (DNA index = DI) which can be used to discriminate and identify different subpopulations of cells and, it yields information of the fractions of cells in the cell cycle phases, whereby treatment induced cell cycle perturbations can be studied. The analysis can be performed on solid tumors or cells in culture. If fine-needle aspirates of solid tumors are used for analysis, several consecutive measurements can be obtained from the same tumor.

In this paper we will review some of our data obtained by flow cytometric DNA analysis in SCCL in patients, hetero-tranplanted to nude mice or in tissue culture. The data illustrate how, by the same method, heterogeneous tumors can be studied intact and complex, or broken down in individual subpopulations grown with or without a host.

2. MATERIALS AND METHODS

DNA analysis was performed by using an integrated set of methods for sample storage, staining and internal standardization. In solid tumors fine-needle aspirates were used for preparation. Samples were stored before analysis by freezing at -80 C (9). The analysis was performed on nuclei isolated by the use of detergent and trypsin, and stained by propidium iodide (10). In some studies a simple, earlier version of the staining method was used (7). Gl-cell DNA content indicated as DI where 1.00 corresponds to the normal human diploid value, was determined by the use of chicken and trout erythrocytes as internal standards, stained and analysed with the sample (11). The flow cytometer used was a FACS III cell sorter (Becton Dickinson, Sunnyvale, CA). The attainable resolution of the DNA analysis is described elswhere (8). The fractions of cells in the cell cycle phases were determined by computer analysis

(1). The details of heterotransplantation and in vitro culture techniques are described elswhere (2,6).

3. RESULTS AND DISCUSSION

Thirty-eight different metastases in 29 consecutive patients with SCCL were examined with a total of 273 fine-needle aspirations. In 23 (79%) only one cell population could be detected. Evidence of two subpopulations with different DI was found in 6 (21%) patients (12). Assessment of the resolution of the analysis led to the conclusion that di- or possibly polyclonality is likely to be higher than 21%.

The treatment-induced cell cycle changes were monitored by consecutive DNA analyses. In one study 14 metastases in 11 patients were monitored during a total of 14 courses of

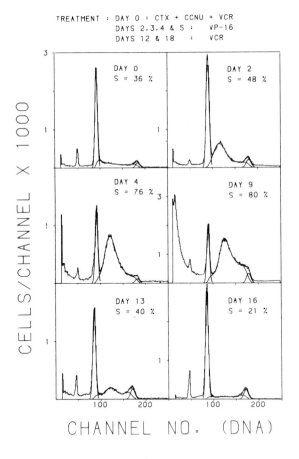

FIGURE 1. DNA distributions obtained by analysis of fine-needle aspirates from a metastasis in a patient with SCCL. The treatment given, and the time of aspiration are indicated.

combination chemotherapy with Cyclophosphamide, CCNU, Vincristine and Methotrexate (13). The cell cycle changes, which
preceded tumor reduction, consisted of a relative decrease in
G1 cells starting on day 1, maximal days 3 to 5. Simultaneously there was an increase in the S-phase. This was
followed in some patients by an increase in G2 + M starting on
day 3, maximal on days 4 to 6. The maximal changes observed in
the cell cycle were: G1, 70% to 1%, S, 32% to 90% and G2 + M,
14% to 88%. The tumor volume changes started on day 2 and were
highly variable, ranging from a brief partial remission (PR)
to a complete remission (CR). The temporary increase in S-
phase cells was more pronounced in the metastases responding
with a CR, than in those responding with a PR. Conversely a

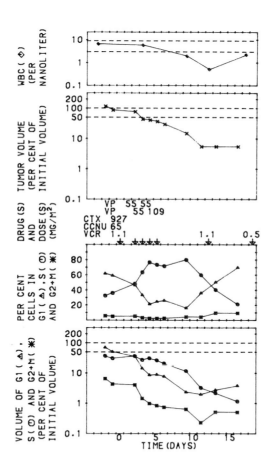

FIGURE 2. The plots show changes in white blood cells (WBC),
tumor volume and the cell cycle, in the same patient as shown
in fig. 1. The plot at the bottom, indicating the volume of
the G1, S and G2 + M compartments, was derived by combining
the information of tumor volume with the cell cycle data.

significant increase in G2 + M cells was found in all
metastases in the PR group whereas only one metastasis in the
CR group exhibited an increase in G2 + M.

An example of the pertubation of the cell cycle that can be
registered by DNA analysis is shown i Fig. 1. The treatment
given in this case was, as indicated on the figure, Cyclophosphamide (CTX), CCNU, VP-16 and Vincristine (VCR). Cells
are arrested in S where an increase from 36% to 80% is
observed. Changes in white blood cell count (WBC) as a measure
of toxicity, and the volume of the metastasis are shown in
Fig. 2, together with the fractions of cells in the cell
cycle, obtained by computer analysis of the histograms shown
in Fig. 1.

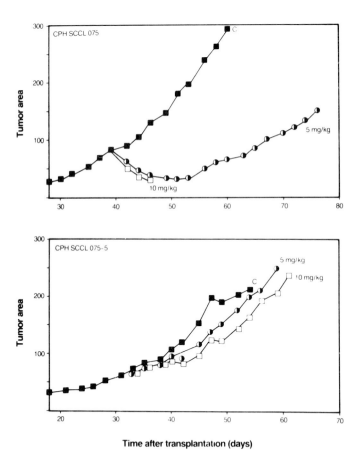

FIGURE 3. Mean growth curves of CPH SCCL 075 and CPH SCCL
075-5 grown in nude mice, and treated with Melphalan in the
doses indicated.

Figures 1 and 2 show considerable cell cycle pertubation and
data like these are potentially useful for early prediction of
sensitivity and thus response, as well as for the design of
treatment schedules seeking exploitation of phase-specific
drug action.

Analysis of cell cycle perturbation data and tumor volume
measurements in patients where 2 different subpopulations were
identified by different DI, indicated that treatment failure
was caused by selection and overgrowth of resistant subpopulations (12,13).

Treatment of patients with SCCL must today, for ethical
reasons consist of combination chemotherapy. It is thus not
known to what extent the individual drugs in a combination
contribute to changes of the type shown in Figs. 1 and 2. More
detailed information of this as well as information of the
sensitivity of different subpopulations from the same tumor,
can be obtained from studies on heterotransplants and in
vitro.

Tumor cells from patients with SCCL have been established as
cell lines in vitro (2). The cell lines or tumor cells taken
directly from patients may be grown as heterotransplants in
nude mice (6). Different subpopulations of heterogeneous
tumors may be separated by cloning in vitro (2) and subpopulations may be examined in tissue culture or as solid tumors
after transplantation to nude mice. An example of this are
results obtained in CPH SCCL 075, a tumor and cell line
established directly from a patient metastasis, and CPH SCCL
075-5, a subpopulation of the former (4).

Fig. 3 shows the growth curves of the tumor in nude mice,
untreated and after single-dose chemotherapy on day 39 with
Melphalan in the doses indicated. It is clear that the parent

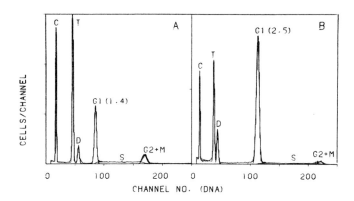

FIGURE 4. DNA distributions of CPH SCCL 075 (A) and CPH SCCL
075-5 (B). The DI of 1.4 and 2.5 were determined by internal
standardization with chicken (C) and trout (T) erythrocytes.

110

tumor (075) is much more sensitive to the drug than the subpopulation (075-5). Flow cytometry was used to identify the
tumors (Fig. 4) CPH SCCL 075 had a DI = 1.4 and CPH SCCL 075-5
a DI = 2.5. Sequential analysis during treatment showed a
marked increase in S-phase cells of the sensitive tumor days
1-6 after treatment (not shown) whereas no change was seen in
the resistant tumor (4).

We have previously shown in Ehrlich ascites tumors that cell
cycle perturbation monitored by flow cytometric DNA analysis
could be used as a test for sensitivity to Adriamycin (3). To
further extend this method to a solid tumor CPH SCCL 075 and
CPH SCCL 075-5 were exposed in vitro for one hour to different

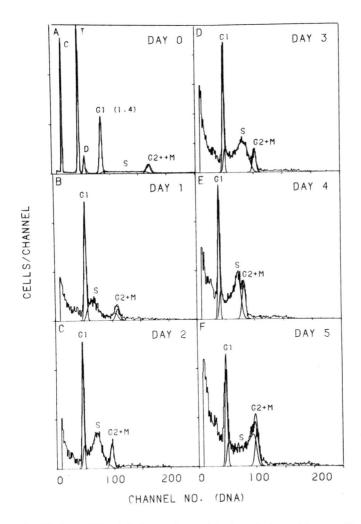

FIGURE 5. DNA histograms obtained in vitro after exposure for
one hour of CPH SCCL 075 to Melphalan, 10^{-3} mg/ml.

concentrations of Melphalan, and the S-phase changes were recorded (5). The results of exposure to 10^{-3} mg/ml are shown in Fig. 5. It is seen that cells are accumulated in and slowly propagate through the S-phase. Only insignificant changes were found in the resistant tumor (5). The similarity between the results shown in Fig. 1 (SCCL in vivo) and in Fig. 5 (SCCL in vitro) is obvious.

4. CONCLUSIONS

1) SCCL is heterogeneous and different subpopulations can be demonstrated by flow cytometric DNA analysis and identified by their DI.

2) Evidence in vivo in patients indicates that treatment failure is caused by selection and overgrowth of resistant subpopulations.

3) Subpopulations of SCCL with different DI may be separated in vitro and grown as heterotranplants in nude mice or in tissue culture.

4) Flow cytometry may be useful for sensitivity testing of tumors.

5) Flow cytometric DNA analysis can be performed equally well in SCCL in patients, in heterotransplanted tumors and in vitro. The analysis is therefore useful for linking results obtained in SCCL grown at different levels of complexity.

REFERENCES

1. Christensen I, Hartmann NR, Keiding N, Larsen JK, Noer H, Vindeløv L: Statistical Analysis of DNA Distributions from Cell Populations with Partial Synchrony. Pulse-Cytometry III. Lutz D. (ed), Ghent: European Press Medicon: 71-78, 1978.

2. Engelholm SA, Spang-Thomsen M, Brünner N, Nøhr I, Roed H, and Vindeløv LL: In Vitro Culturing of Tumor Cells on Soft Agar. In: SE Salmon, IM Trent (eds) Human Tumor Cloning p. 197-203. Grune & Stratton, 1984.

3. Engelholm SA, Spang-Thomsen M, Vindeløv LL: A Short-term in Vitro Test for Tumour Sensitivity to Adriamycin Based on Flow Cytometric DNA Analysis. Br. J. Cancer 47: 498-502, 1983.

4. Engelholm SA, Spang-Thomsen M, Vindeløv LL and Brünner N: Effect of Melphalan on Growth Curves and Cell Cycle Distribution of Four Human Small Cell Carcinomas of the Lung Grown in Nude Mice. (Submitted)

5. Engelholm SA, Spang-Thomsen M, Vindeløv LL, and Brünner N:
    Chemosensitivity of Human Small Cell Carcinoma of the Lung
    Detected by Flow Cytometric DNA Analysis of Drug-induced
    Cell Cycle Perturbations in Vitro. (Submitted)

6. Spang-Thomsen M, Nielsen A, Visfeldt J: Growth Curves of
    Three Malignant Tumors Transplanted to Nude Mice. Exp.
    Cell Biol. 48: 138-154, 1980.

7. Vindeløv LL: Flow Microfluorometric Analysis of Nuclear
    DNA in Cells from Solid Tumors and Cell Suspensions.
    Virchows Arch. B Cell Path. 24: 227-242, 1977.

8. Vindeløv LL, Christensen IJ, Jensen G, Nissen NI: Limits
    of Detection of Nuclear DNA Abnormalities by Flow Cyto-
    metric DNA Analysis. Results Obtained by a Set of Methods
    for Sample-Storage, Staining and Internal Standardization.
    Cytometry 3: 332-339, 1983.

9. Vindeløv LL, Christensen IJ, Keiding N, Spang-Thomsen M,
    Nissen NI: Long-Term Storage of Samples for Flow Cyto-
    metric DNA Analysis. Cytometry 3: 317-322, 1983.

10. Vindeløv LL, Christensen IJ, Nissen NI: A Detergenttrypsin
    Method for the Preparation of Nuclei for Flow Cytometric
    DNA Analysis. Cytometry 3: 323-327, 1983.

11. Vindeløv LL, Christensen IJ, Nissen NI: Standardization of
    High-Resolution Flow Cytometric DNA Analysis by the
    Simultaneous Use of Chicken and Trout Red Blood Cells as
    Internal Reference Standards. Cytometry 3: 328-331, 1983.

12. Vindeløv LL, Hansen HH, Christensen IJ, Spang-Thomsen M,
    Hirsch FR, Hansen M, Nissen NI: Clonal Heterogeneity of
    Small-Cell Anaplastic Carcinoma of the Lung Demonstrated
    by Flow-Cytometric DNA Analysis. Cancer Res. 40: 4295-
    4300, 1980.

13. Vindeløv LL, Hansen HH, Gersel A, Hirsch FR, Nissen NI:
    Treatment of Small-Cell Carcinoma of the Lung Monitored by
    Sequential Flow Cytometric DNA Analysis. Cancer Res 42:
    2499-2505, 1982.

CLINICAL APPLICATIONS OF THE BIOLOGIC PROPERTIES OF SMALL CELL LUNG CANCER

DESMOND N.CARNEY

1. INTRODUCTION

Small Cell Lung Cancer (SCLC) accounts for approximately 20-25% of all new cases of primary lung cancer. Unlike the other major forms of lung cancer (collectively referred to as Non-SCLC (NSCLC), SCLC is highly sensitive to both chemotherapy and radiation therapy. However, while major advances have been made in the treatment of SCLC with up to 90% of patients demonstrating a response to combination chemotherapy and radiation therapy and between 5-10% of patients achieving long term survival (i.e. > 2 years), results have plateaued over the past 5 years (1). While many factors may influence response to therapy and survival including extent of disease at diagnosis, physiologic or performance status of the patient, it is also possible that therapeutic responses observed may be related to properties inherent within the tumour cells themselves. These differences could represent expression of drug or radiation resistance genes, or genes coding for more malignant behaviour such as cellular oncogenes.

The recent advances in tissue culture techniques, in particular the development of a highly selective serum-free hormone supplemented medium (HITES) (2), has greatly improved our ability to establish continuous cell lines of SCLC. In a recent report cell lines of SCLC were successfully established from 72% of 41 tumour-containing specimens (3). The ability to reproducibly grow tumour cells in vitro from the majority of SCLC patients has permitted a detailed evaluation of the biological characteristics of these tumour cells. In this Chapter the properties of SCLC cells will be described and contrasted with other types of lung cancer and their application in the management of patients with SCLC will be discussed.

2. CELL LINE ESTABLISHMENT

The detailed techniques used to establish cell lines of lung cancer have been previously described (3). In brief, specimens for culture were obtained from a variety of organ sites including bone marrow, lymph node aspirates and biopsies, malignant effusions, and surgically resected tumour masses. For most specimens containing tumour cells the time to "establishment" of a cell line ranged from 3-6 months. At that time cells demonstrated continued growth and ease of ability to passage cells at a low cell density. The nature of these cultured tumour cells have been evaluated by gross morphology, cytology, nude mice tumorigenicity, growth properties, and the expression of a variety of biomarkers and peptides. Results obtained with SCLC cells were compared with these of Non-SCLC lung cancer lines and a variety of other human tumours. The results of these studies discussed below are based on the detailed analysis of 50 cell lines of SCLC, 19 cell lines of Non-SCLC lung cancer, and 18 non lung tumour cell lines.

3. BIOMARKER EXPRESSION IN LUNG CANCER CELL LINES

All cell lines were evaluated for the expression of the key APUD enzyme L-dopa decarboxylase (DDC,EC41.1.28), the APUD marker neuron specific enolase (NSE,EC4.2.11), the peptide bombesin (BL1), and the BB isozyme of creatine kinase (CK-BB,EC2.7.3.2.)using previously described
methods (3-7). Significant differences in the expression of these 4 biomarkers between SCLC and NSCLC lung cancer cell lines were observerd
(Table 1). While expression of these biomarkers was usually higher in
established SCLC specimens in contrast to fresh biopsy specimens,analy-
sys of DDC and CK-BB in fresh specimens of SCLC and NSCLC also confirmed
the differences in the expression of these markers in these cell types.
The demonstration of differences in the expression of biomarkers between
SCLC and NSCLC may have practical application in the subtyping of different types of lung cancer, in particular anaplastic or poorly differentiated tumours. Such distinction would have a major impact on therapy
selection and prognosis. For patients with NSCLC hope for cure and long
term survival depends upon the ability to surgically resect the primary
tumour. In contrast for patients with SCLC, hope for cure is dependent
upon the sensitivity of the tumour to systemic cytotoxic therapy.

TABLE 1. Markers which distinguish small cell from non-small cell lung
cancers

Biomarker	SCLC	Non-SCLC
L-dopa Decarboxylase	++	-
Bombesin	++	-
Neuron Specific Enolase	++	-
Creatine Kinase BB	++	-
HLA Expression	-	++
Leu-7 Antilgen	++	-
Peptide Hormones	++	-

In addition to the analysis of fresh specimens for DDC and CK-BB, the
expression of both NSE and BL1 in cells has been evaluated using monoclonal antibodies and immunohistochemical techniques. While individual
cell heterogeneity may be observed in SCLC tumours in their expression
of these markers, preliminary data suggests that such immunohistochemical techniques may be of value in the subtyping of SCLC and NSCLC. Whether clinical differences are observed between tumours with different
antigenic expression remains to be determined and should be evaluated in
prospective studies of lung cancer therapy. Several investigations have
recently reported on the value of serum and cerebrospinal fluid analysis
of various biomarkers including NSE and CK-BB in the management and staging of patients with SCLC (8-12) (Table 2). In studies of large numbers
of newly diagnosed patients with SCLC, serum NSE was raised in 65-73%
of all patients including 39-59% of patients with limited stage disease
and up to 87% of patients with extensive stage disease. In contrast
elevated levels of serum NSE were detected in only 11% of patients with
other histologic types of lung cancer (9). Mean levels of NSE were
significantly higher in patients with extensive disease compared with
levels in patients with limited stage disease. Like many other markers
in SCLC, elevated serum levels did not correlate with metastatic disease

in a specific site including brain, bone marrow, liver etc. No differences in overall response rate or survival was observed among patients with limited disease who initially had a normal or raised NSE level. In all studies serial NSE determinations showed an excellent correlation between serum NSE and clinical response (8-10). In the study by Johnson et al a rise in serum NSE was detected in 15 of 23 patients (65%) as many as 12 weeks before clinical evidence of relapse could be detected. These data suggest that serum NSE determinations may be useful in the staging of patients with SCLC in monitoring response to therapy, and may help predict the recurrence of disease before it is otherwise clinically detected (Table 2).

TABLE 2. Serum Neuron Specific Enolase Determination in Patients with Small Cell Lung Cancer

No. Patients	No. + Elevated NSE	Stage of Disease		Ref.
		Limited	Extensive	
94	65 (69%)	15/38 (39%)	49/55 (87%)	8
20	13 (65%)	-	-	9
93	68 (73%)	23/39 (59%)	45/54 (85%)	10

Creatine Kinase (EC2.7.3.2) occurs in large amounts in the serum primarily as 3 isozymes; CK-BB which is found in large amounts in the brain, gastro intestinal tract and genitourinary tract; CK-MM which is found in skeletal muscle and cardiac muscle, and the hybrid CK-MB, which is found primarily in cardiac muscle. In healthy adults the predominant serum isoenzyme is CK-MM and the concentration of serum CK-BB is very low. In a recent study of 105 newly diagnosed SCLC patients elevated serum CK-BB was detected in 26%, including 1 of 42 patients with limited stage disease and 26 (41%) of these with extensive stage SCLC.
After adjusting for the number of metastatic sites detected, survival among patients with a normal pretreatment CK-BB was significantly better than in patients with an elevated CK-BB ($p < 0.001$) (Median 13 months versus 5 months). Like other markers sequential serum determinations revealed an excellent correlation between response to therapy and serum CK-BB (12).
While these data on serum NSE and CK-BB determinations in SCLC patients suggest that their measurement may be of value in the management of patients with this disease, like many other serum components which have been proposed as "biomarkers" of SCLC or as indicators of the extent of diagnosis etc. (such as ACTH, Calcitonin, CEA), at the present time it appears that none seem either sensitive or specific enough to mandate their widespread use either in the management of patients with lung cancer, or in screening for early detection.
CNS metastases occur with symptoms in 30% of patients with SCLC. Routine screening with scans etc. are of limited value. The development of new techniques for early diagnosis of these lesions would be of major clinical importance. Recently Pedersen et al (13) showed that CSF levels of vasopressin were significantly elevated in patients with metastases. While the overall value of measurement of biomarkers in the CSF is unclear prospective studies in SCLC patients will define their role.

4. HETEROGENEITY IN BIOMARKER EXPRESSION IN SMALL CELL LUNG CANCER: CLASSIC AND VARIANT SCLC.

Although there are signficant differences in the expression of DDC, BLI, NSE and CK-BB between SCLC and non-SCLC it has recently been recognized that considerable heterogeneity exists in the expression of these biomarkers within cell lines of small cell lung cancer (3, 14, 15). Based on the expression of these markers SCLC cell lines can be subdivided into two major groups, namely classic and variant (Table 3). Classic cell lines which account for 70% of SCLC lines all express significantly elevated levels of the key APUD enzyme DDC. In contrast variant cell lines have undetectable or very low levels of this enzyme. In addition to DDC, Classic cultures have elevated levels of BLI, NSE and CK-BB. Variant cultures have undetectable levels of BLI in addition to DDC, but continue to express elevated levels of both NSE and CK-BB (3,15). The presence of elevated levels of CK-BB in both classic and variant SCLC cultures can clearly differentiate cell of SCLC origin from those of non-SCLC which have very low or undetectable levels of this enzyme. Of interest, there is an excellent correlation in SCLC cultures between the expression of an elevated DDC, and the presence of neurosecretary granules on electron microscopy examination (3).

TABLE 3. Comparison of the Biological properties of Classic and Variant Cultures of Small Cell Lung Cancer

Characteristic	Classic	Variant
Morphology	Type 1 & 11	Type 111 & 1V
Histology	SCLC	SCLC/LC
Neurosecretery Granules	Present	Absent
L-DDC	Elevated	Absent
BL1	Elevated	Elevated
NSE	Elevated	Elevated
CK-BB	Elevated	Elevated
Cloning Efficiency	2.5%	13%
Doubling Time	72 hrs.	32 hrs.
Radiation Sensitivity	Sensitive	Resistant
C-myc Amplification	No	Yes
Peptide Hormones	Common	Absent

5. GROWTH PROPERTIES OF CLASSIC AND VARIANT SCLC CELLS

Although the majority of SCLC cell lines grow as floating aggregates of cells, gross differences between cell lines can be detected in cultures. Based on their gross appearances SCLC cells can be subdivided into 4 main subgroups: Type 1 & 11 grow as very-tight to tightly packed aggregates of floating cells which frequently demonstrate central necrosis, Type 111 cell lines grow as very loosely attached floating aggregates of cells while Type 1V SCLC cell lines grow as attached monolayer cultures. Of interest there is an excellent correlation between the gross appearances of the cells and their biochemical profile. Among 37 cell lines with Type 1 & 11 morphology 33 (88%) were classic cell lines (3). In contrast, of 13 cell lines with a Type 111 & 1V morphology, 11 (85%) belonged to the variant class of SCLC. As the in vitro appearances can be typed within several days of plating a fresh specimen in culture, it may be possible to predict the phenotype (classic or variant) of the cultured cells at that time.

Cytologically and histologically cultured cells resemble the tumour cells in the original biopsy specimens. The majority of classic SCLC cultures exhibit features typical of the intermediate cell type of SCLC (3,15).In addition to morphological differences classic and variant cell lines exhibit significant differences in their growth rate and in vitro radio sensitivity (3,15,17). Variant cultures of SCLC have a significantly shorter doubling time (32v71 hrs.); and a higher cloning efficiency in agarose (13 v 2%) than classic cultures.When inoculated into athymic nude mice variant cultures have a shorter period to tumour formation than classic cultures. Using standard in vitro techniques several groups have reported on the in vitro radiobiological properties of classic and variant SCLC cultures (16,17). The results of these studies indicate that variant cultures exhibit a marked increase in radiation resistance in vitro compared to classic cultures. In addition, following a 200 rad dose (a fraction commonly used in treating lung cancer patients) variant cultures demonstrated a 2-5 fold increase in survival compared to classic cultures.

5. ONCOGENE STUDIES IN SMALL CELL LUNG CANCER
   The more "malignant" behaviour in vivo and in vitro of variant cultures compared to classic cultures has prompted studies of the expression of oncogenes in SCLC cells (18,19). In a detailed study of 35 cell lines C-myc amplification (20-80 fold) was noted in 7 of 9 variant cell lines. In contrast only one of 24 classic cell lines had amplification of the gene. In amplified variant cell lines, significant expression of C-myc RMA was also observed. These oncogene abnormalities were found in early passage cultures suggesting they had occurred in the patient. Karyologic studies of these C-myc amplified lines revealed homogeneously staining chromosomal regions (17). These"HSR's"do not necessarily correlate to the original location of the amplified gene and may also differ in chromosome location between tumours.

More recently a second oncogene abnormality, amplification of N-myc has been observed in several cell lines of SCLC. Increased expression and / or amplification of this C-myc related gene N-myc had previously been demonstrated in neuroblastomas and retinoblastomas (19,20). Indeed among patients with neuroblastomas amplification of N-myc is associated with a more advanced clinical stage and prognosis. In addition to detecting N-myc amplification/expression in several established cell lines similar oncogene abnormalities were identified in tissues harvested from fresh biopsy specimens. The amplification of N-myc is often associated with the appearance of double minute chromosomes. The finding of increased myc-related gene amplification or expression in many SCLC cell lines, and in patients specimens, and in particular in the variant type of SCLC, suggests that these genes may play an important role in the transition of low malignant SCLC ("classic") to the highly malignant variant phenotype. The development of monoclonal antibodies against myc oncogene products and their use in vivo and in vitro may help to clarify the role of these oncogenes in the progression of SCLC.

6. PEPTIDE HORMONE EXPRESSION IN CULTURES OF SMALL CELL LUNG CANCER.
   Among patients with lung cancer paraneoplastic syndromes are most frequently observed in patients with SCLC. In studies of cell lines

peptide hormone secretion is most frequently observed in SCLC cells in
contrast to cell lines of non SCLC (21,24) Peptides frequently detected
in SCLC cell lines include bombesin, calcitonin, AVP, lyotropin, neurotensin and ACTH(22). Peptides such as metencephalin, gastrin, VIP and
substance P are rarely detected in SCLC cell lines (22). Among cell
lines of SCLC lineage, peptide secretion was less frequently observed
in variant compared to classic cultures. The presence of many peptide
hormones in SCLC suggests that they may have a physiologic role in this
tumour type. The amphibian neuropeptide bombesin, a 14 amino acid peptide,
is expressed in high amounts in classic SCLC cultures and is actively
secreted by these cells into their culture medium. In addition a single
class of high affinity receptors for bombesin have been identified on
some SCLC cells which are similar to those previously described in non-
tumours (25). The addition of exogeneous bombesin to SCLC in vitro can
stimulate the clonal growth and DNA synthesis of SCLC cells in vitro(26).
These data suggest that bombesin may function for SCLC cells and suggest
that the growth of this tumour type in vivo may be altered by interfe-
ring with the binding of bombesin to its cellular receptor.

7. ANTIGENIC EXPRESSION OF SMALL CELL LUNG CANCER CELLS
   Many investigators have developed and characterised monoclonal antibodies with high specificity for both SCLC and non-SCLC (27,30). Such
reagents have been used in the detection and typing of lung cancer cells
in clinical specimens using immunohistochemical staining techniques.
While considerable heterogeneity exists in antigenic expression both in
individual tumours and between tumours from different patients, studies
are underway to determine if differences in antigenic expression are of
prognostic importance.
More recently Doyle et al (31) has demonstrated that the major Class 1
histocompatibility antigens HLA and B2 microglobulin are expressed at
easily detectable levels in non-SCLC cells, but are either not expressed
or expressed at very low levels in SCLC. Using molecularly cloned
probes for HLA and B2M, southern blot analysis showed the genes to be
intact at the DNA level. However, Northern blot analysis showed that
in most cases HLA and B2M nRNA was not expressed or expressed at much
lower levels in SCLC. Of interest and as has been shown in other
tumour systems, incubation of SCLC cells with gamma interferon lead to
the development of detectable amounts of HLA and B2M on their cell surface.
More recently several investigators have demonstrated that SCLC cells
express antigens more commonly detected on a variety of haematopoetic
cells including monocytes, natural killer (NK) cells and lymphocytes
(32, 33). Using the anti-Leu 7 monoclonal antibody Bunn et al (33)
showed that an antigenic determinent present on NK cells is also expressed on SCLC cells, their putative precursor cells, and other benign and
malignant neuroendocrine tumours. In contrast this antigen is rarely
detected on NSCLC cells. Thus, like Class 1 histocompatibility antigens,
it appears that the Leu 7 antigen may be used clinically to distinguish
SCLC from NSCLC.

8. SUMMARY
   The ability to establish and characterise cell lines of lung cancer
has greatly improved our understanding of the biological properties
of these tumours. It is clear from the above data that not only are there
clear differences in the properties of SCLC and NSCLC, but indeed

considerable heterogeneity exists among cell lines of SCLC. Detailed studies of SCLC cell lines indicates that at least two major categories exist, classic and variant cell lines. As variant cells have a more "malignant" behaviour in vitro it is likely that clinical correlations of this phenotype exists. Recent reports have reported that patients with SCLC who on histologic examinations have a mixed small cell/large cell morphology have a significantly worse prognosis than patients with "pure" SCLC (34). The recognition that some variant cell lines have been established from patients with this mixed morphology, and that the variant cells are more "aggressive" in behaviour suggests that variant lines are the in vitro correlation of the mixed SC/LC morphology.

This accumulation of biological data on SCLC indicates the heterogeneity of this tumour and implies that SCLC is a spectrum of diseases with different behaviour and prognosis. As the biological properties appear to be clinically important future clinical studies in the management of SCLC patients should include the evaluation of biological properties as part of the initial staging and work-up of patients with this disease.

REFERENCES

1. Morstyn G, Ihde DC, Lichter AS, Bunn PA, Carney DN, Glatstein E and Minna JD: Small cell lung cancer 1973-1983: Early progress and recent obstacles. Int J Rad Oncol 10:515-539,1984.
2. Carney DN, Bunn PA, Gazdar AF, Pagan JA, Minna JD: Selective growth in serum-free hormone supplemented medium of tumor cells obtained by biopsy from patients with small cell carcinoma of the lung. Proc Natl Acad Sci USA 78:3185-3189,1981.
3. Carney DN, Gazdar AF, Bepler G, Guccion J, Moody TW, Marangos PJ, Zweig HM and Minna JD: Establishment and identification of small cell lung cancer cell lines having classic and variant features. Cancer Res In press 1985.
4. Baylin SB, Abeloff MD, Goodwin G, Carney DN and Gazdar AF: Activities of L-dopa decarboxylase and diamine Oxidase (histaminase)in human lung cancers and decarboxylase as a marker for small (oat) cell cancer in cell culture. Cancer Res 40:1990-1994,1980.
5. Marangos PJ, Gazdar AF and Carney DN: Neuron specific enolase in human small cell carcinoma cultures. Cancer Lett 15:67-71,1982.
6. Moody TW, Pert CB, Gazdar AF, Carney DN and Minna JD: High levels of intracellular bombesin characterises human small cell lung carcinoma. Science, 214:1246-1248,1981.
7. Gazdar AF, Zweig HM, Carney DN, Van Steirteghen AC, Baylin SB and Minna JD: Levels of creatine kinase and its BB isoenzyme in lung cancer specimens and cultures. Cancer Res 41: 2773-2777,1981.
8. Carney DN, Marangos PJ, Ihde DC, Bunn Jr PA, Cohen MH, Gazdar AF and Minna JD: Serum neuron-specific enolase: a marker for disease extent and response to therapy of small cell lung cancer. Lancet, 583-585, 1982.
9. Ariyoshi Y, Kato K, Ishiguro Y et al.: Evaluation of serum neuron specific enolase as a tumour marker for carcinoma of the lung. Gann 74:219-225,1983.
10. Johnson D, Marangos PJ, Forbes JT et al.:Potential utility of serum neuron specific enolase in small cell carcinoma of the lung. Cancer Res 44:5402-5414, 1984.

11. Vinores SA, Bonnin JM, Rubinstein LJ and Marangos PJ: Immunohistoche-
    mical demonstrations of neuron specific enolase in neoplasms of the
    CNS and other tissues. Arch Pathol Lab Med 108: 536-540,1984.
12. Carney DN, Ihde DC, Zweig MH, Cohen MH and Gazdar AF: Serum Creatine
    Kinase BB in small cell lung cancer. Cancer Res 44:5399-5403,1984.
13. Pedersen AG, Hammer M, Hansen M and Sorenson PS: Cerebrospinal fluid
    vasopressin as a marker of central nervous system metastases from
    small cell bronchogenic cancer. J Clin Oncol 3:48-53,1985.
14. Gazdar AF, Carney DN, Russel EK, Simms HL, Baylin SB, Bunn PA Jr,
    Guccion JG, Minna JD: Small cell carcinoma of the lung: establishment
    of continuous clonable cell lines having APUD properties. Cancer Res
    40:3502-3507,1980.
15. Gazdar AF, Carney DN, Nau M and Minna JD: Characterization of variant
    subclasses of cell lines derived from small cell lung cancer having
    distinctive biochemical, morphological and growth properties. Cancer
    Res in Press 1985.
16. Carney DN, Mitchell JR, Kinsella TJ: In vitro radiation and chemo-
    sensitivity of established cell lines of human small cell lung cancer
    and its large cell variants. Cancer Res 43:2806-2811,1983.
17. Goodwin G and Baylin SB: Relationships between neuro endocrine differ-
    entatiation and sensitivity to radiation in culture line OH-1 of
    human small cell lung carcinoma. Cancer Res 42:1361-1367,1982.
18. Little DD, Nau MM, Carney DN, Gazdar AF, Minna JD: Amplification and
    expression of the C-myc Oncogene in human lung cancer cell lines.
    Nature 306:1984-196,1983.
19. Nau MM, Carney DN, Battey J, Johnson B, Little C, Gazdar AF, Minna JD:
    Amplification, expression and rearrangement of C-myc and N-myc onco-
    genes in human lung cancer. Curr Top Microbiol Immunol 113:172-177,
    1984.
20. Brodeur GM, Seeger RC, Schwab M et al.: Amplification of N-myc in
    untreated neuroblastomas correlates with advanced stage. Science
    224:1121-1124,1984.
21. Sorenson GD, Pettengill OS, Brinck-Johnsen T, Cate CC and Maurer LH:
    Hormone production by cultures of small-cell carcinoma of the lung.
    Cancer, 47:1289-1296,1981.
22. Gazdar AF, Carney DN, Becker KL, Deftos L, Go VL, Marangos PJ,
    Moody TW, Wolfsen AR and Zweig MH: Expression of peptide and other
    markers in lung cancer cell lines. Recent Res Cancer Res,In press
    1984.
23. Goedert M, Reeve JG, Emson PC and Bleehen NM: Neurotensin in human
    small cell lung carcinoma. Br J Cancer 50:179-183,1984.
24. Moody TW, Carney DN, Korman LY et al.: Neurotensin is produced by
    and secreted from classic small cell lung cancer cells. Life
    Science 36:1727-1732,1985.
25. Moody TW, Bertness V, Carney DN 1983a: Bombesin-like peptides and
    receptors in human tumor cell lines. Peptides 4:683-686.
26. Cuttitta F, Carney DN, Mulshine J, Moody TW, Fedorko J, Fischler A,
    Minna JD: Bombesin-like peptides can function as autocrine growth
    factors in human small cell lung cancer. Nature (in press),1985.
27. Cuttitta F, Rosen S, Gazdar AF and Minna JD: Monoclonal antibodies
    which demonstrate specificity for several types to human lung cancer
    Proc Natl Acad Sci USA,78:4591-4595,1981.
28. Rosen ST, Mulshine JL, Cuttitta F, Fedorko J, Carney DN, Gazdar AF,
    Minna JD.1984: Analysis of human small cell lung cancer differentia-
    tion antigens using a panel of rat monoclonal antibodies: A common

link between small cell lung cancer, endodermal tumours and neuro-blastoma. Cancer Res. 44:2052-2061.

29. Mulshine JL, Cuttitta F, Bibro M, Fedorko J, Farigon S, Little C, Carney DN, Gazdar AF, Minna JD, 1983: Monoclonal antibodies that distinguish non-small cell from small cell lung cancer. J Immunol 131:497-502.

30. Baylin SB, Gazdar AF, Minna JD, Bernal SD and Shaper JH: Aunique cell-surface protein phenotype distinguishes human small cell from non-small cell lung cancer. Proc Natl Acad Sci,79:4650-4654,1982.

31. Doyle LA, Martin JW, Funa K, Gazdar AF, Carney DN, Martin SE, Linnoila I, Cuttitta F, Mulshine J, Bunn PA, Minna JD: Markedly decreased expression of Class 1 histocompatability antigens,proteins, and mRNA in human small cell lung cancer. J Exp Med 1985.

32. Lipinski M, Braham K, Cailland JM, Carley C, Tursz T: HNK-1 antibody detects an antigen expressed on neuroectodermal cells. J Exp Med 158:1775-1780.

33. Bunn PA Jr, Linnoila I, Minna JD, Carney DN, Gazdar AF: Small cell lung cancer, endocrine cells of the fetal bronchus, and other neuro-endocrine cells express the Leu-7 antigenic determinant present on natural killer cells. Blood 65:764-768,1985.

34. Radice PA, Matthews MJ, Ihde DC, Gazdar AF, Carney DN, Bunna PA, Cohen MH, Fossieck BE, Makuch RW, Minna JD: The clinical behaviour of mixed small cell/large cell bronchogenic carcinoma compared to pure small cell subtypes. Cancer 50:2894-2902,1982.

PEPTIDE HORMONES IN LUNG CANCER

C.GROPP

1. INTRODUCTION
   In patients with small cell lung cancer a number of peptide hormone
immunoreactive proteins have been demonstrated by radioimmunoassay
(1 - 3).
In some cases lung tumors of this histological type are associated with
paraneoplastic syndromes caused by the peptide hormone production of the
tumor. On the basis of these and some other biological criteria of the
small cell lung tumors (S.C.C.) it was suggested that these tumor cells
might be derived from pulmonary endocrine cells, the Kultschitzky-like
cells in the bronchial submucosa. In vivo and in vitro results suggested
that the secretion of calcitonin and bombesin are specific for small
cell lung tumors (4 - 6).
Immunohistological demonstration of calcitonin and other peptide hormones
in small cell as well in non-small cell lung tumor cells done in our group
were in contradiction to this concept(7). (Table 1)

TABLE 1. Demonstration of peptide hormones in paraffin sections of lung
         tumor tissues by the immunoperoxidase technique (positive/number
         of investigated tumors)

Carcinoma	ACTH	ß-Lipotropin	ß-Endorphin	Alpha-MSH	Calcitonin	ß-HCG
"Oat cell"	18/36	9/36	3/36	3/19	3/36	7/36
Squamous	12/21	7/21	4/21	4/13	2/21	10/21
Large cell	10/19	6/19	1/19	3/10	3/19	9/19
Adeno	3/ 5	1/ 4	0/ 4	1/ 3	1/ 4	1/ 4
Total	43/81	23/80	8/80	11/45	9/80	27/80

To answer the question whether all lung tumors produce a variety of
peptide hormones, 30 permanent and more than 60 primary tumor cell cultures
were established from pleural and pericardial exudates or wedge biopsies
from human bronchocarcinoma. Peptide hormones were determined in the
culture medium of these cell lines and were isolated for further characterization.

2. ESTABLISHMENT OF LUNG TUMORS IN CELL CULTURE AND NUDE MICE
The successful establishment of continuous cell lines from
SCC has been reported by Pettengill et al.(8) and by
Gazdar et al. (9). Some of the described cell lines
produced peptide hormones, which could be demonstrated in the
cell culture media. Stimulated by these studies, we have
established a number of hormone-producing lung cancer cell
lines in culture and as xenotransplants in nude mice. Long
term cell lines were established from small cell, large cell,
squamous and adeno lung tumors (WHO-classification). Small cell
lung tumor cell lines were derived from malignant effusions,
cell cultures of the other tumors originated from surgical
biopsies. Most of the cell lines were set up by direct cloning
of disintegrated tumor tissue in MEM Dulbecco's or RPMI 1640
medium containing 16,6% fetal calf serum. ACTH, calcitonin,
salmon-like calcitonin, bombesin and neurotensin were
determined by commercial radioimmunoassays in the culture
medium.
For xenotransplantation cell suspensions from permanent cell
lines were injected s.c. into athymic nude mice (NMRI). All
handling of mice took place in a laminar flow hood. Mice were
maintained in sterile plastic cases in a standard animal room
(37°C, 70% humidity of the atmosphere). Once tumors reached a
size greater than 4 cm^3, they were transplanted into nude mice
or prepared for cell culture and histological examinations.
The characteristics of some cell lines are given in table 2.

3. PEPTIDE HORMONE PRODUCTION IN CELL CULTURE
The permanent cell lines established until now have their
origin in 6 small cell, 5 large cell, 9 squamous and 5 adeno
carcinoma of the lung. These lines hav been stable for 12-14
months. In vivo secretion of ACTH, bombesin, calcitonin and
neurotensin has been demonstrated for lung tumor cells
belonging to the major different 4 histological types. (Fig. 1)

FIGURE 1.
Peptide hormones
secreted into
the culture
medium by
various tumor
cell lines

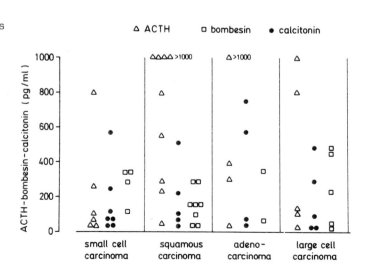

TABLE 2. Characteristics of small cell and non-small cell lung cancer cell lines

Lung cancer cell line		Origin	Doubling time(days) in culture	Doubling time(days) in culture	Start of tumor growth in mouse after injection of 1×10^7 cells (days)	Hormones produced
Small cell carcinoma	MR-22	Pleural fluid	4	2- 7	14	Bombesin, calcitonin, neurotensin, estriol
	MR-55	Lung biopsy	5			ACTH, bombesin, calcitonin, neurotensin
	MR-86	Pleural fluid	4	1- 2	7	-
Squamous carcinoma	MR- 9	Lung biopsy	1.5			ACTH, bombesin, neurotensin
	MR-25	Lung biopsy	1	20	80	ACTH, bombesin, calcitonin, neurotensin, substance P
	MR-32	Lung biopsy	1.5	6- 12	70	Bombesin, calcitonin, substance P
Adeno-carcinoma	MR- 5	Lung biopsy	1-3	20	140	ACTH, bombesin, β-lipotropin
	MR-13	Lung biopsy	6			ACTH, bombesin, calcitonin, neurotensin
Large cell carcinoma	MR- 8	Lung biopsy	3	6-10	35-42	ACTH, bombesin, calcitonin, CSF, β-lipotropin, neurotensin

126

Observing all cell cultures established, long term and short
term cultures, positive ACTH levels were found in 31% of the
cell cultures deriving from small cell, 30% from large cell,
24% from squamous and 20% from adeno carcinoma of the lung.
Bombesin production was observed in 50% of small cell, 60% of
large cell, 63% of squamous and 46% of the adeno lung tumor
cell cultures. Elevated calcitonin levels were demonstrated in
culture media of 43% of small cell, 50% of the large cell,
20% of squamous and 39% of the adeno carcinoma cell cultures.
Neurotensin positivity was determined in 25% of the small cell,
40% of the large cell, 20% of the squamous and 30% of the adeno
lung tumor cell cultures. Additionally we were able to
demonstrate in long term cell cultures of all 4 histologies
salmon-calcitonin-like activity.

FIGURE 2.Salmon- and
human calcitonin
secreted into the
culture medium by
various tumor cell
lines.

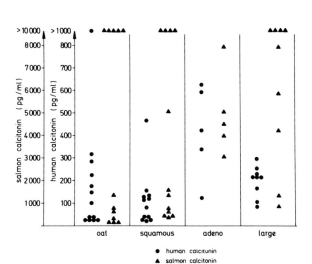

4. ISOLATION AND CHARACTERIZATION OF PEPTIDE HORMONES

Calcitonin-immunoreactive protein
    Recently we described the separation of three calcitonin-
immunoreactive proteins from sera of patients with small cell
lung cancer by means of gel filtration techniques (10).
        These proteins, with molecular weights of 100.000,
48.000 and 20.000 daltons, were degradable by incubation with
sodium dodecyl sulfate under reducing conditions to a 17.000-
dalton protein; this is relatively stable and might be a
calcitonin prohormone synthesized by the tumor cells.
To confirm these results and for further characterization of
the tumor calcitonin we started in vitro studies with
calcitonin-producing lung tumor cell lines.
Calcitonin-containing culture medium was lyophilized and
subjected to gel chromatography on AcA 54 (LKB Stockholm,
Sweden) columns. By this method three calcitonin-immuno-

reactive protein fractions with molecular weights of 100.000,
50.000 and 20.000 daltons were identified in the medium of
SCLC, but also of NSCLC cell lines. These high-molecular-
weight calcitonin fractions correspond to the calcitonin
proteins isolated in former studies from sera of patients with
SCLC. There was no difference between calcitonin proteins from
SCLC and NSCLC cultures, and no protein with the molecular
weight of physiological calcitonin was detectable.
In further experiments the different calcitonin fractions were
incubated in the presence of sodium dodecyl sulfate and then
separated by electrophoresis on 10% polyacrylamide gels. The
denaturation of the various fractions resulted in a 17.000-
dalton calcitonin-immunoreactive band. An additional 3.400-
dalton calcitonin appeared on the gels, which has a molecular
weight similar to that reported for physiological calcitonin.
The calcitonin-immunoreactive proteins were further
characterized by their behavior on ion-exchange chromatography.
Most of the 20.000-dalton calcitonin fraction was bound to
DEAE-Sephacel at neutral pH and low conductivity and could be
eluted at slightly acid pH in the presence of 55mM NaCl. The
100.000-dalton fraction did not interact with DEAE-Sephacel.
Affinity chromatography on concanavalin A-Sepharose and lentil
lectin-Sepharose showed that the calcitonin-immunoreactive
proteins did not contain any glycoprotein component with
alpha-D-mannosyl or sterically related residues. To investigate
the stability of the calcitonin fractions against proteolytic
degradation they were incubated for different times in the
presence of trypsin. This procedure resulted in a degradation
of the 100.000- and 50.000-dalton calcitonin-immunoreactive
protein to a relatively stable 17.000-dalton protein. This
17.000-dalton protein seems to be a relatively stable core-
protein, which may represent the calcitonin prohormone
synthesized by the lung tumor cells. Preliminary studies with
C-cell carcinoma cell lines indicate that the calcitonin-
immunoreactive protein from lung cancer cell lines is bio-
chemically different from the calcitonin synthesized by C-
cell carcinoma cells (Luster et al., to be published).

5. ACTH-IMMUNOREACTIVE PROTEIN

In patients' sera the ACTH levels are relatively low as
ACTH is highly sensitive to proteolytic activities. Therefore,
direct separation of ACTH-immunoreactive material from sera by
gel filtration is impossible. For isolation and characterization of this peptide hormone it is beneficial to establish
hormone-producing cell lines. In addition, we have devised
a method for further enrichment of the ACTH-immunoreactive
material by way of affinity chromatography on Cibacron Blue
F3GA followed by lyophilization. After this step, gel
filtration resulted in four ACTH-immunoreactive peaks, of more
than 100.000, 30.000, 20.000 and 4.500 daltons. The two major
peaks also showed immunoreactivity with ß-lipotrophin, which
probably derives from the same precursor molecule as ACTH
(Gropp et al. 1983). Our results also show that like
calcitonin, ACTH is also synthesized both from SCLC and from
NSCLC cell lines. After the establishment of several ACTH-
secreting lung tumor cell lines and methods for the isolation

and enrichment of this peptide hormone
further studies for the characterization of ACTH-immunoreactive proteins are under way. Table 3 gives a brief
summary of the characteristics of the calcitonin and ACTH
synthesized by our cell lines.

TABLE 3. Characterization of calcitonin and ACTH immunoreactive proteins from serum and tissue of lung tumor patients
as well as from culture medium of permanent cell lines

Immuno-reactivity	Molecular weight determined by gel filtration	Protein A affinity chromatography	Lectinchromatography
Calcitonin	100,000 48,000 20,000	No interaction with immunoglobulins	No glycoprotein component
ACTH	100,000 30,000 20,000 4,800	Binding of IgG	Glycoproteincomponent

Immuno-reactivity	Ion exchange chromatography	SDS stability	Stability against proteolytic activities	Isoelectric point
Calcitonin	Specific enrichment of the 20,000-dalton fraction	Degradation to 17,000-dalton core protein	17,000-dalton protein most stable	5.5−6.0
ACTH	No interaction	No longer measurable by immunological methods	Labile	−

6. INFLUENCE OF PEPTIDE HORMONES ON TUMOR CELL PROLIFERATION
    The role of the peptide hormones for growth and function of
the hormone-producing cells themselves, i.e. an autocrine or
paracrine role, is of great interest. For example, a lung
tumor cell line, BEN, has been described, which produces
calcitonin and has calcitonin receptors (11)
our laboratory we started investigations of the influence of
physiological human hormones on the proliferation and biosynthetic activities of lung tumor cells. In these experiments
small cell and non-small-cell lung tumor cultures were
incubated in the presence of hormone-containing medium, and
cell proliferation was measured by incorporation of radiolabeled thymidine in to the DNA. The results are shown in
Fig. 3. Not only the proliferation but also the hormone
production of some cell lines was increased by incubation of

the cultures with human hormones (12).

FIGURE 3. Influence of
peptide hormones and
other biological active
substances (I, insulin;
T, transferrin;
S, selenium) on the
proliferation of lung
tumor cells in vitro

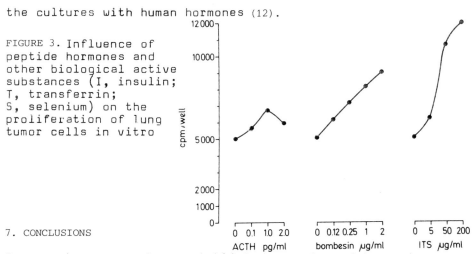

7. CONCLUSIONS

In recent years we have established a number of hormone-
producing cell lines from SCLC. These cell lines can secrete
various peptide hormones into the culture medium simultaneously. Beside SCLC cell lines, several cell lines from NSCLC have
been cultured in our laboratory. These cell lines also
produce various peptide hormones and no difference in the
hormone profile has been detected in comparison with the SCLC
cell lines. For example, we have three ACTH-producing adenocarcinomas, and the cell line with the highest calcitonin
secretion is also well characterized as an adenocarcinoma. In
addition, bombesin, a peptide hormone believed to be highly
specific for SCLC, has been demonstrated in some squamous
and adenocarcinoma cell lines. These results suggest that
lung tumors of all histological types are able to synthesize
peptide hormones. This hypothesis is also supported by earlier
immunohistological studies on lung tumor tissues, in which we
were able to demonstrate ACTH, calcitonin, and ß-lipotrophin
in nearly 50% of NSCLC tumors (7). Our studies
on the isolation and characterization of calcitonin and ACTH
secreted from lung cancer tumor cells showed a relatively
stable calcitonin-immunoreactive protein with a molecular
weight of 17.000 daltons and ACTH-immunoreactive proteins with
molecular weights of more than 100.000, 30.000, 20.000 and
4.500 daltons.
These results lead to the conclusion that lung tumor cells
synthesize an ACTH and a calcitonin prohormone, which are
secreted by the tumor cells after incomplete intracellular
degradation. Finally, cell proliferation of SCLC and NSCLC
cell lines have been stimulated in vitro by peptide hormones.
Further studies will show whether these peptide hormones
might act as growth factors for lung tumor cells.

REFERENCES

1. Silva OL, Becker KL, Primack A, Doppman I, Snider RH: Ectopic secretion of calcitonin by oat-cell carcinoma. N Engl J Med 290: 1122-1124, 1974.
2. Horai I, Nishihara H, Tateishi R, Matsuda M, Hattori S: Oat-cell carcinoma of the lung simultaneously producing ACTH and serotonin. J Clin Endocrinol Metab 27:212-219, 1973.
3. Ratcliffe JG, Podmore J, Stack BHR, Spilg WGS, Gropp C: Circulating ACTG and related peptide in lung cancer. Brit J Cancer 45:230,1982.
4. Roos BA, Lindall AW, Baylin SB, O'Neill JA, Frelinger AL, Birnbaum RS, Lambert PW: Plasma immunoreactive calcitonin in lung cancer. J Clin Endocrinol Metab 50:659-666,1980.
5. Silva OL, Broder LE, Doppman JL, Snider RH, Moore CF, Cohen MH, Becker KL: Calcitonin as a marker for bronchogenic cancer. Cancer 44: 680-684,1979.
6. Moody TW, Pert CB, Gazdar AF et al: High levels of intracellular bombesin characterize human small cell lung carcinoma. Science 214:1246-1248,1981.
7. Gropp C, Sostmann H, Luster W, Kalbfleisch H, Lehmann FG, Havemann K: ACTH, β-lipotropin,β -endorphin, β -HCG, calcitonin and CEA in lung tumor tissues. In: CEA und andere Tumormarker, Uhlenbruck Wintzer, Tumor Diagnostik-Verlag,Leonberg,pp 217-226,1981.
8. Pettengill OS, Faulkner CS, Wurster-Hill DH et al.: Isolation and characterization of a hormone-producing cell line from human small cell anaplastic carcinoma of the lung. JNCI 58:511-518,1977.
9. Gazdar AF, Carney DN, Russell EK et al: Establishment of continuous clonable cultures of small cell carcinoma of the lung which have amine precursor uptake and decarboxylation cell properties. Cancer Res 50:3502-3507,1980.
10. Luster W, Gropp C, Sostmann H, Kalbfleisch H, Havemann K: Demonstration of immunoreactive calcitonin in sera and tissues of lung cancer patients. Europ J Cancer Clin Oncol 18:1275-1283,1982.
11. Ham J, Ellison ML, Lumsden J: Tumor calcitonin: Interaction with specific calcitonin receptor. Biochem J 190:545-550.
12. Luster W, Gropp C, Havemann K: Peptide hormone synthesizing lung tumor cell lines: Establishment and first characterization of biosynthetic products. Acta Endocr Supp 253:24-25,1983.

MECHANISMS OF ONCOGENESIS

A.J. VAN DER EB

1. INTRODUCTION

The idea that cancer arises from somatic mutations in cellular genes was recently confirmed when it was discovered that point mutations can activate normal genes so that they will become cancer genes or oncogenes. While it has often been assumed that cancer results from a loss of essential functions by mutation, the recent discoveries have demonstrated that at least some forms of cancer are generated as a result of mutational activation of genes which results in the production of dominant cancer genes.

This new concept arose from studies in which DNA isolated from human or animal tumors was introduced into suitable tissue culture cells (usually NIH 3T3 cells, an established cell line derived from NIH Swiss mouse embryos). These DNA transfection studies revealed that some of the tumor DNAs were capable of inducing oncogenic transformation in 3T3 cells, whereas DNA from normal cells or tissues did not show this property. The genes responsible for this transforming activity in 3T3 cells were identified by the use of recombinant DNA techniques and they often turned out to be identical or related to cellular genes that had just been discovered to be the cellular homologues of viral oncogenes. Since oncogenic RNA viruses have played a central role in the discovery of cellular transforming genes or cellular oncogenes, the properties of this group of viruses will be briefly discussed.

2. THE ONCOGENES OF TUMORIGENIC RETROVIRUSES ARE DERIVED FROM THE GENOME OF ANIMAL CELLS

Oncogenic RNA viruses belong to the group of the retroviruses, i.e. they have the unique property that they can convert their single-stranded RNA genome into a double-stranded DNA copy. This DNA copy integrates into the host cell genome and then functions as the intermediate in the production of progeny virus. These viruses can be divided into 2 groups on the basis of their tumorigenic potential: (1) The slow leukemia viruses, which can induce leukemias or lymphomas after a long latency period (± 6 months or longer) and (2), the acute leukemia and sarcoma viruses which induce cancer after much shorter latency periods.

The former group of viruses contains genomes with 3 genes, designated gag, pol and env. These genes code for viral structural proteins and for the enzyme reverse transcriptase (pol), but none of the genes appears to be an actual transforming (onco-)gene. The genome is flanked by identical nucleotide sequences, called LTRs (Long Terminal Repeats), which contain the signals required for the regulation of the expression of gag, pol and env. The oncogenic potential of this group of viruses is caused, in some cases at least, by the activity of the LTRs and not by viral protein products. When a DNA copy of a retrovirus happens to integrate close to

Table 1. Examples of acute RNA tumor viruses and possible functions of their oncogenes

Virus	Oncogene	Function of cellular oncogenes
Rous sarcoma virus (chicken)	src	Tyrosine kinase; (inner face of plasma membrane). Role in growth factor-induced signal transduction.
Avian myelocytomatosis virus (chicken)	myc	Activation of gene expression? (nuclear). Control of cell proliferation
Avian erythroblastosis virus (chicken)	erb-A	–
	erb-B	Receptor for epidermal growth factor (EGF) (plasma membrane)
Harvey murine sarcoma virus (rat)	H-ras	GTP-binding proteins; GTPase-activity ("G-proteins"?) (inner face of plasma membrane). Role in growth factor-induced signal transduction
Kirsten murine sarcoma virus (rat)	K-ras	
Abelson murine leukemia virus (mouse)	abl	Tyrosine kinase (associated with plasma membrane)
FBJ murine osteosarcoma virus (mouse)	fos	Biochemical function unknown (nuclear) Control of cell proliferation
Simian sarcoma virus (monkey)	sis	One of the chains of platelet-derived growth factor (PDGF)

certain cellular oncogenes (see below), one of the LTRs can activate such a gene and this can result in oncogenic transformation.

The acyte RNA tumor viruses are derived from the slow leukemia viruses and they differ from this group in that they contain novel nucleotide sequences that are not related to any of the genes of the slow leukemia viruses. These novel sequences had been inserted at random positions in the genome of the slow leukemia viruses and this was accompanied by deletions in the viral genome. Studies with mutants of acute RNA tumor-viruses have shown that this new genetic information was in fact respon-sible for the acute transforming potential of the viruses, and these sequences were therefore called oncogenes. Surprisingly, further studies have shown that these oncogenes were not true viral genes but were derived from the genome of the cells in which the parental slow viruses had replicated. Thus, the oncogene of the Rous sarcoma virus (RSV), which is called v-src, also occurs as a cellular gene (c-src) in chicken cells, the host cell of RSV and related leukemia viruses. Interestingly, c-src not only occurs in chicken and bird cells, but also in mammalian cells, in fact in the genomes of all vertebrates, and even in invertebrates. The c-src gene is also expressed in normal cells and tissues. These results together indicate that src is a gene that is highly conserved in evolu-tion and fulfils an essential function. Basically similar results have been obtained for other v-oncogenes: they occur in many or all verte-brates and sometimes in invertebrates and often, but not always, they are expressed as RNA and protein. Table 1 shows a number of examples of acute RNA tumor viruses and their oncogenes.

3. WHY DO VIRAL ONCOGENES CAUSE CANCER ?

An obvious question is why these oncogenes will cause cancer when they are part of a viral genome, whereas they apparently fulfil normal functions in animal cells. A possible answer to this question was suggested by the observation that the v-src gene in RSV-transformed cells is expres-sed at a much higher level than is the c-src gene in normal cells. The interpretation could then be that the overexpression of an oncogene can cause a normal cell to become a tumor cell. To test this possibility, several cellular oncogenes, which had been isolated by means of recombi-nant DNA techniques from normal human or animal cells, were reintroduced into non-transformed cells. The oncogenes were either supplied with their own promoter (the regulatory elements for expression) or with heterologous promoters which were known to have a strong inducing potential for gene expression. The introduction of e.g., a c-H-ras gene with its own promoter into NIH 3T3 cells did not result in transformation but the introduction of the same gene linked to a viral LTR (which contains a rather strong promoter) caused oncogenic transformation. This experiment demonstrated that indeed overexpression of a normal cellular oncogene can cause trans-formation. Subsequent experiments with other oncogenes, however, showed that overexpression does not always lead to transformation, but that alterations in or around the oncogene may also be required for the activa-tion (see below).

4. CELLULAR ONCOGENES ARE INVOLVED IN NON-VIRALLY INDUCED CANCER

The discovery of cellular homologues of the viral oncogenes led to the question of whether these genes play a role in spontaenous, non-virally induced cancer. To answer this Weinberg and his colleagues isolated DNA from human tumors or from cancers chemically-induced in animals, and transfected the DNAs by means of the "calcium technique" to cultures of

NIH 3T3 cells. These cells were known to be suitable for assaying the transforming activity of certain viruses and viral nucleic acids. The results of these experiments showed that DNA from certain tumors indeed was capable of inducing transformation in the 3T3 cells. The transformed cells were also oncogenic and formed tumors in nude mice. By means of recombinant DNA techniques it was shown that the gene responsible for the transforming activity of a human bladder tumor DNA was identical to the cellular H-ras gene. (The mammalian genome contains 3 ras genes, H-ras, K-ras and N-ras. The former two had already been identified as the oncogenes of acute rat sarcoma viruses, but the latter (N-ras) so far has not been found in a retrovirus). The results, therefore, showed that a cellular homologue of a viral oncogene can indeed be involved in spontaneous cancer.

The question arises "Why can the bladder carcinoma ras gene induce oncogenic transformation whereas the corresponding ras gene from normal human tissue does not have this property?"This was answered by the use of artificially constructed DNA molecules consisting of a normal H-ras allele in which defined parts were substituted by the corresponding parts of the bladder carcinoma gene. These studies showed that the introduction of DNA segments containing sequences coding for the N-terminal end of the carcinoma ras protein were able to convert the normal gene into a transforming gene. Further studies showed that the oncogenic activity was brought about by a single point mutation resulting in the substitution of the 12th amino acid, glycine, into valine. Apparently, the substitution of a single amino acid in the ras protein is sufficient to modify its properties so that it becomes an oncogene. Subsequent studies in numerous other laboratories have shown that about 15-20% of human or animal tumor DNAs had transforming activity in NIH 3T3 cells and that in the majority of the cases studied a ras gene was responsible for the transforming activity. The activation of the ras genes was caused by point mutations resulting in substitution either of the 12th amino acid or of the 61st amino acid of the ras protein, and sometimes the 13th amino acid. Why most of the tumor DNAs fail to cause transformation in 3T3 cells is not known. It is possible that the negative tumor DNAs do not contain activated ras genes but carry mutations in other genes which do not cause transformation in 3T3 cells. Alternatively, they may contain activated ras genes, but activation is so weak that it is difficult to detect in 3T3 cells. (It is known that certain amino acid substitutions result in weakly transforming ras genes).

5. CANCER CELLS MAY CONTAIN MORE THAN ONE ACTIVATED ONCOGENE

A number of observations suggested that oncogenic transformation may involve the activation of more than one oncogene. Three examples suggesting that two oncogenes are activated in cancer cells will be mentioned here: (1). The leukemic cell line HL60, which is derived from a human promyelocytic leukemia, was known to contain an amplified c-myc gene. C-myc is an oncogene that was first discovered in the avian leukemia virus MC29. The gene was amplified 20-30 fold, which resulted in the elevated expression of myc RNA and protein, suggesting that myc may be responsible for the leukemic state of the cells. Analysis of the transforming activity of DNA isolated from HL60 cells in the 3T3-assay gave a positive reaction, i.e. transformed foci were observed, but the transforming gene turned out not to be c-myc but N-ras. Yet, there was evidence indicating that the high expression of myc also contributed to the transformed state of the cells. This was suggested by the observation that treatment of HL60 cells with the vitamin D3 derivative 1,25 (OH)$_2$D3 or with retinoic acid resulted

in the inhibition of c-myc expression, which was followed by differentiation into either granulocytes or monocytes (1). These effects are reversible and this shows that the elevated myc expression almost certainly
plays a role in the oncogenic phenotype of the cells.
(2). Burkitt lymphoma is a human tumor derived from B-lymphoid cells. The
tumor cells are characterized by specific chromosome translocations,
usually involving the translocation of a segment of the long arm of
chromosome (chr.) 8 to the long arm of chr.14, and vice versa. The
translocation point at chr.8 is located very close to the site of the
c-myc gene, and the translocation point at chromosome 14 always occurs
within the region coding for the immunoglobulin heavy chains. As a result
of the translocation, the myc gene is usually transferred to chr. 14, to a
site within the Ig^H region. Probably as a result of its association with
the Ig^H genes the myc gene is expressed at an elevated level, or at least
is continuously (or constitutively) expressed. The myc gene is normally
only active during the differentiation of pre-B cells to immunoglobulin-
producing cells and it is shut off in mature plasma cells. Burkitt lympho-
ma$_H$ cells produce continuously large amounts of immunoglobulin, hence the
Ig^H genes are in an active state. This may be the reason why the translo-
cated myc gene (as opposed to the non-translocated myc allele) is also
active: it has come under the influence of the active Ig^H domain. When the
DNA from Burkitt cells was tested in the 3T3 assay, again N-ras was found
to be activated, which suggests that two oncogenes are involved in the
generation of the Burkitt tumor.
(3). As has been discussed above, NIH 3T3 cells can be transformed by
activated ras oncogenes. In contrast, primary cultures of rodent cells
(e.g. rat embryo or baby rat kidney) can not be stably transformed by
activated ras. The 3T3 cells differ from primary cells in that they have
acquired an unlimited lifespan, and thus are "immortalized". In contrast,
primary rat embryo cells have a limited life span, unless they are conver-
ted to an immortalized state, either spontaneously or as a result of viral
or carcinogen-induced transformation. When primary rat embryo cells were
transfected with an activated ras gene plus an activated myc gene (i.e. a
myc gene regulated by an LTR) full transformation to oncogenic cells was
obtained. Thus, activated myc is needed to convert the primary cells to a
3T3 cell-like state, which shows again that two activated oncogenes are
needed to transform a normal cell to a tumor cell.
    Whether more than two oncogenes are involved in spontaneous cancer is
not known. It is possible that progression of tumor cells to more highly
malignant states or acquisition of metastatic properties may involve a
third category of oncogenes.

6.THE MECHANISM OF ACTIVATION OF ONCOGENES AND THEIR ROLE IN CARCINOGENESIS
    The mechanism by which oncogenes are activated is not known exactly.
Point mutations in ras genes are probably caused by errors during repair
of DNA damage or during semi-conservative DNA replication. How myc genes
are activated is completely obscure (gene translocation or gene amplification) and it is even unknown whether myc activation can be induced
directly by carcinogenic agents or is caused by other factors.
    Little information is available either on the role of activation of
myc and ras genes in the process of oncogenesis: is myc always activated
first, followed by ras, or vice versa? Some studies have indicated that
ras activation may occur at late stages of oncogenesis. For example, a
human melanoma was found to lack detectable ras oncogene activity in the
3T3 assay, but some of the metastases derived from it did contain an

activated ras gene (2). On the other hand, ras activation could already be detected in benign papillomas (3), suggesting that it may occur also at early stages of oncogenesis.

As to the specificity of ras genes for certain tumors again no clear correlations have been found between types of tumors and types of activated ras genes. There is some specificity for the activation of N-myc (an oncogene related to c-myc) in neuroblastoma and certain types of lung carcinoma, and for the activation of N-ras in hematopoietic tumors. Recently, experimental evidence has been obtained by Barbacid and co-workers (personal communication) that some carcinogens induce specific tumors in rats and mice, and that each type of tumor (induced by a particular agent) carries a particular activated ras gene. For example, the carcinogen NMU induced lymphomas in mice in which only N-ras is activated, and mammary carcinomas in rats in which H-ras is activated; DMN induced kidney carcinomas in rats in which K-ras is activated, etc. The causes for this specificity are unknown. It is conceivable that there is a relationship with an increased activity of particular ras genes in certain organs or tissues at the time of exposure to the carcinogen and that highly active genes are more accessible to carcinogens than less active genes. It is also possible that the carcinogens tend to accumulate in such organs or tissues, increasing the chance that mutations occur in ras genes.

7. FUNCTIONS OF CELLULAR ONCOGENES

Relatively little information is available on the natural functions of cellular oncogenes. Recent studies have indicated that at least some oncogenes have a role in cellular growth and differentiation. This was suggested by the following observations: the oncogene sis represents the gene coding for one of the chains of platelet-derived growth factor, PDGF, a growth hormone required for proliferation of fibroblastic cells; erb-B is derived from the gene coding for the receptor of epidermal growth factor, EGF, a receptor found on a large variety of cells. Stimulation of quiescent cells with PDGF leads to a rapid and transient increase in the expression of two oncogenes, fos (after about 20 min) and myc (after 2-4 hours). Furthermore, there is evidence to indicate that the oncogenes src, ros and probably ras all have a natural role in the transmission of signals induced by growth factors when they bind to their receptors. Normal cellular oncogenes (a better name would be proto-oncogenes) can be activated to cancer genes either by mutation of the oncogene product itself (as in the case of ras genes) or by a change in the vicinity of the oncogene which results in a loss in its ability to be regulated by other genes or signals (e.g. c-myc in Burkitt cells). Mutational activation could cause a gene product to be constantly, or longer than normal, in its active form, so that it can transmit signals along the signal transmission pathway also when it is not stimulated to transmit signals. Oncogene activation can also be caused simply by the turning-on of the expression of a gene, e.g. of a gene coding for a growth factor such as PDGF. (See also Table 1).

As will be clear from this summary, the discovery of oncogenes represents an important breakthrough in cancer research which will hopefully enable us to unravel eventually the molecular basis of cancer. Our knowledge is still very fragmentary, however, and much more work is needed to obtain a complete understanding of the mechanism(s) of carcinogenesis.

REFERENCES

The following review articles contain detailed information on the subjects discussed in this paper.

Bishop J.M. Cellular oncogenes and retroviruses Ann.Rev.Biochem. 52(1983) 301-354.

Varmus, H.E. The Molecular genetics of cellular oncogenes. Ann.Rev.Genet. 18(1984)553-612.

References cited in the text:
1. Reitsma, P.H. et al. Regulation of myc expression in HL60 leukemia cells by a vitamin D metabolite. Nature 306(1983)492-494.

2. Albino, A.P. et al. Transforming ras genes from human melanoma: a manifestation of tumor heterogenicity? Nature 308(1984)69-74.

3. Balmain, A. et al. Activation of the mouse cellular Harvey-ras gene in chemically induced benign skin papillomas. Nature 307(1984)658-660.

ADHESION MECHANISMS IN LIVER METASTASIS

E. ROOS

1. INTRODUCTION

The liver is a major target organ for metastasis formation by many tumor types, including lung carcinoma (1). The aim of the present study is the elucidation of mechanisms underlying the interactions between tumor cells and liver cells, which lead to the incorporation of a tumor cell into liver tissue, and thus enable the formation of a metastatic tumor. The approach was, first, to observe by electron microscopy the invasion of tumor cells into the intact liver, both in vivo and perfused in situ; second, to isolate liver cells and to reproduce the interactions that had been observed in vivo, by addition of tumor cells to short-term cultures of these liver cells; and third, by perturbing the in vitro interactions mainly by antibodies directed against either the tumor cells or the liver cells. The studies in vivo indicated that the invasion mechanism was qualitatively comparable for different tumor cell types although large quantitative differences were seen particularly between, on the one hand, diffusely infiltrating lymphoma cells and, on the other hand, tumor cell types which gave rise to nodular metastases. In contrast, the in vitro experiments clearly showed that at the molecular level mechanisms were quite distinct, particularly for lymphoma as compared to carcinoma cells.

2. THE INTACT LIVER

Invasion into the intact liver was studied by electron microscopy on sections prepared from mouse livers in which tumor cells had been arrested at various time intervals before fixation. We used mainly livers that were perfused in situ with a medium to which the tumor cells were added (2,3), but also livers from mice injected intraportally in vivo (2-5).   .

Virtually all tumor cell types were 100% efficiently arrested in the liver capillaries. The cells breached the endothelium by extension of multiple small protrusions into (and not often between) the endothelial cells. The latter cells apparently responded by formation of channels through which the protrusions could reach the extravascular space (figs. 1,2). Since liver capillaries are largely devoid of basement membrane, these protrusions were not impeded to make contact with the underlying epithelial cells, the hepatocytes.   .

Subsequently, some extended psuedopods enlarged and deeply intruded the hepatocyte layer (2,3). The end result of this process was the incorporation of the tumor cell into this layer (fig.3). Close contact between the hepatocyte and tumor cell surface and folding of thin hepatocyte cytoplasmic extensions around the tumor cells suggested active interaction and strong adhesion between the two cell types. The described sequence of

140

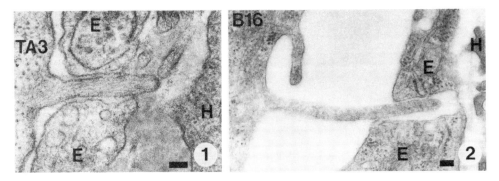

Figs. 1 & 2. Breaching of liver endothelium by tumor cells. Fig. 1: TA3 mammary carcinoma, fig. 2: B16 melanoma. Protrusions are extended through openings formed within endothelial cells (E). H: hepatocyte. Bar: 0.1 um.

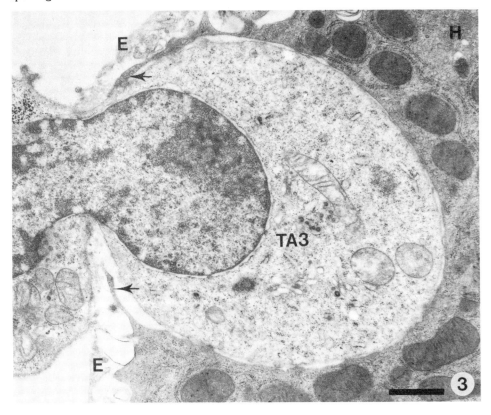

Fig. 3. Invasion of the liver by TA3 mammary carcinoma. Note folding of hepatocyte (H) around the tumor cell. E: endothelium. Bar: 1 um.

events was qualitatively similar for various tumor cells, but quantitatively the cells differed quite extensively. Lymphomas sometimes invaded massively, resulting in large numbers of tumor cells distributed diffusely throughout the liver tissue. In contrast, comparatively few cells of melanomas, carcinomas and some lymphomas invaded, resulting in a limited number of nodular metastases. Many of the latter cells did extend protrusions through the endothelium. In contrast, the next step, the intrusion of large pseudopods into the hepatocyte layer, was rarely seen.

3. IN VITRO CULTURES
3.1. Endothelial cells

Liver sinusoidal endothelial cells were isolated from collagenase-dispersed rat livers, and were maintained in culture for up to 24 hours. These cells were characterized by their extensive networks of fenestrations and tended to reconstitute their in situ morphology (6). Highly invasive lymphoma cells adhered to these cultured endothelial cells and in the presence of some rat serum even tended to become encircled by the endothelial cells, suggesting strong interaction (fig.10). In contrast, low-invasive lymphoma and carcinoma cells did not adhere (6). Since these tumor cells are efficiently arrested in the liver, it would seem that arrest is due to the small diameter of the capillaries rather than adhesion to the endothelium. As will be discussed below, adhesion to endothelium may be one of the factors determining the invasiveness, particularly of lymphoma cells (see section 4.1).

3.2. Hepatocytes

Rat hepatocytes were also isolated after collagenase perfusion. After 24h in culture, these cells form monolayers that are morphologically reminiscent of intact liver. Tumor cells added to the cultures adhered to the exposed hepatocyte surface (7). Highly invasive lymphoma cells subsequently invaginated at a hepatocyte boundary, moved between the liver cells, and accumulated under the monolayer (fig.4). Within 4-5 hours extensive invasion was seen, and after 24 hours virtually all cells were located within the monolayer (fig.5).

Carcinoma cells also adhered to hepatocytes (fig.6). Some cells invaded the monolayer (fig.7) but this process was rather slow and involved relatively few cells (7). Microtubule-disrupting drugs such as colchicin strongly enhanced invasion (8). Observations of serial sections led to the conclusion that invagination did not always take place at a hepatocyte boundary but that instead the upper surface of a single hepatocyte was often indented. This was never seen with the lymphoma cells and suggested that the mechanism of interaction might be different for these two tumor cell types (7).

4. EFFECT OF ANTIBODIES
4.1. Polyclonal antibodies

To identify the cell surface molecules involved, we have prepared antibodies inhibiting the described interactions. These antibodies were raised against the tumor cells as well as against liver plasma membrane subfractions, enriched in either the hepatocyte contiguous surface or the sinusoidal surface.

142

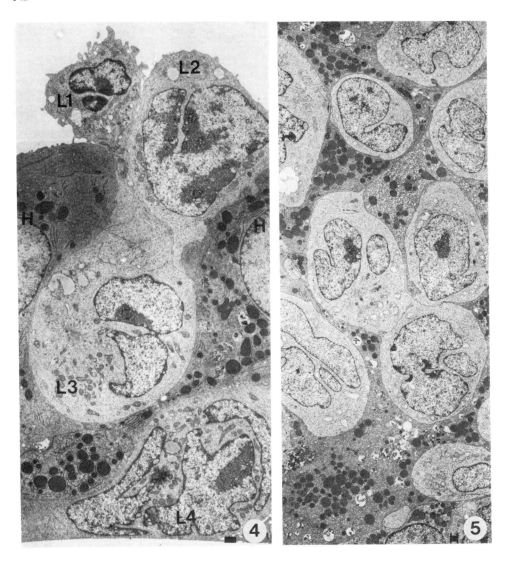

Fig. 4. Invasion of MB 6A lymphosarcoma cells (L1-L4) into a hepatocyte (H) culture. L1 and L2 are still on the upper surface of the culture, but have started to invade between the hepatocytes. L3 has already been incorporated in the monolayer, and L4 is located between hepatocytes and substrate where ultimately all lymphosarcoma cells accumulate. Bar: 1 um.

Fig. 5. Section through a hepatocyte monolayer, parallel to the substrate, 24 h after addition of MB 6A lymphosarcoma cells. The tumor cells are distributed diffusely, similar to what is seen in the intact liver. Bar: 1 um.

Some rabbit antisera against sinusoidal face membranes were found to contain inhibitory antibodies (9,10). Some antisera inhibited only the adhesion of lymphoma cells and others only adhesion of the carcinoma cells (10). Antibodies raised against the tumor cells, in the form of monovalent Fab fragments, also inhibited adhesion, again specific for either cell type (9, and unpublished results). Since adhesion was also differentially sensitive to the presence of Mg-ions (10) and adhesion of lymphoma, but not carcinoma cells was strongly inhibited by microtubule- disrupting agents such as colchicin (8), it became evident that the surface molecules as well as the cellular machinery involved was quite distinct for lymphoma as compared to carcinoma cells (10).

Antibodies against contiguous face-enriched membranes slightly inhibited the adhesion of lymphoma cells to the exposed hepatocyte surface but had more effect on the subsequent invasion between the hepatocytes, quite in contrast to antibodies against the sinusoidal surface (9). Furthermore, adhesion but not subsequent invasion was inhibited by anti-lymphoma antibodies. This suggested that the two steps in the invasion process: initial adhesion and subsequent invasion were mediated by distinct surface molecules, as illustrated in fig.8 (11).

Antibodies against purified endothelial cells interfered with adhesion of lymphoma cells not only to endothelial cells but also to hepatocytes, suggesting that on both liver cell types a similar molecule is involved. This led us to propose the model depicted in fig.9 (11). This model was based on the consideration that strong adhesion to the luminal surface in situ would lock the cells in the vessel and thus prevent rather than enhance invasion. However, if the adhesion molecule involved would be predominantly present at the extravascular surface, pseudopods would be able to anchor at that surface enabling them to pull themselves through the endothelial opening. Lack of adhesion to the endothelial surface might be one of the reasons why this pseudopodal extension, and therefore invasion of the liver, is comparatively rare in case of carcinoma cells.

4.2. Monoclonal antibodies

Adhesion molecules can be identified by their ability to neutralize the inhibitory effect of polyclonal antibodies. This requires extensive purification of surface proteins while maintaining their neutralizing activity. This procedure is attempted for some of the described antibodies but has proven to be quite cumbersome. An alternative approach is to raise monoclonal antibodies which allow for the direct identification of the involved adhesion molecule. We have as yet obtained one such antibody, designated OPAR-1 (12), reacting with the hepatocyte surface and inhibiting the adhesion of carcinoma cells. Adhesion of lymphoma cells is not impeded by OPAR-1, affirming our previous conclusions about the specificity of this interaction. The antigens detected by OPAR-1 have molecular weights of 125 and 100 kDa and are abundantly present on the hepatocyte surface but not on endothelial cells, in line with our observation that carcinoma cells do not adhere to liver endothelium. Outside the liver the antigen is only found in the skin, so that its role in metastasis is likely to be restricted to the liver. For reasons discussed elsewhere (12) we suspect that the OPAR-antigen is related to (pro)collagen.

144

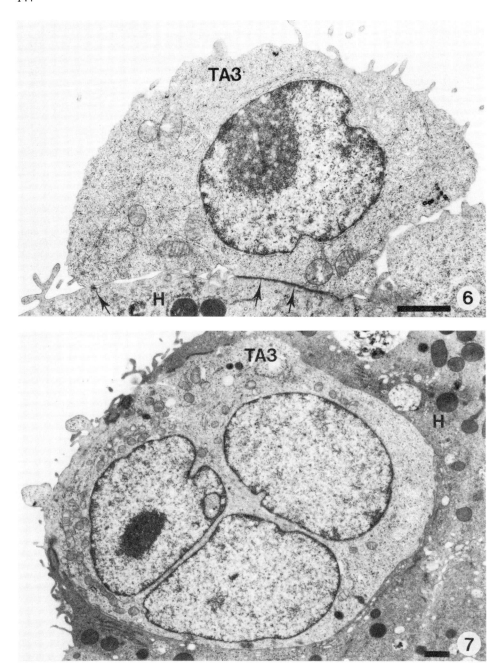

Fig. 6. Adhesion of TA3 mammary carcinoma cell to cultured hepatocyte
(H). Note formation of junctions (arrows). Bar: 1 um.
Fig. 7. Deep invagination of a cultured hepatocyte by a TA3 mammary car-
cinoma cell, 24 hours after addition of the tumor cells. Bar: 1 um.

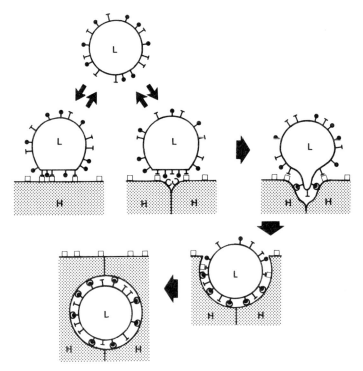

Fig. 8. Model for invasion of lymphoma cells into hepatocyte cultures. Weak reversible adhesion to exposed surface is mediated by other surface molecules than adhesion to contiguous surface necessary for invasion.

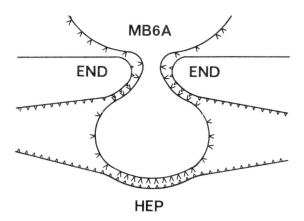

Fig. 9. Model for passage through endothelium. Pseudopod adheres to extra-vascular surface of endothelium and to hepatocytes, possibly via the same surface molecule, and is thus enabled to pull itself out of the vessel.

5. T-CELL HYBRIDOMAS

As described in previous sections, certain lymphomas are extraordinarily invasive. This might be due to the expression of the invasion potential exhibited by normal lymphoid cells in certain stages of maturation. For instance, activated T-lymphocytes invade hepatocyte monolayers in much the same manner as malignant lymphoma cells (13). To test this notion we have fused activated T-lymphocytes with non-invasive and non-metastatic T-lymphoma cells and found that the resulting T-cell hybridomas were highly invasive and upon i.v. injection were highly metastatic, most extensively to the liver but also to kidneys, ovaries, spleen and lymph nodes (14). This shows that properties of normal cells, when expressed in appropriate tumor cells may enhance malignancy. We have also shown that such fusion and acquisition of invasive properties can occur spontaneously in vivo (15), but it is as yet uncertain whether this may also happen in humans.

6. HUMAN TUMOR CELLS

As yet, we have mainly used mouse tumors. The interactions with rat liver cells were essentially similar to those with mouse cells indicating lack of species specifity. Moreover, we have now also found that human carcinoma (fig.11) and certain lymphoma cells invade rat hepatocyte cultures in much the same way as their murine counterparts (unpublished). Thus, human tumor cell surface molecules involved in liver metastasis formation, may be identified using the rat liver cell cultures. In particular, we hope that the production of monoclonal antibodies will be easier than in case of murine cells because of the supposedly higher antigenity of the human adhesion molecules in mice and rats.

7. CONCLUSIONS

We conclude that cellular interactions involved in liver metastasis formation are much more complex than originally thought based on the in vivo observations. In particular, our results point to the involvement of many different cellular molecules, and to considerable specificity both with regard to tumor cell type and to target tissue. However, we have so far seen no differences between various carcinomas tested. Thus, although we have not worked with lung carcinoma cells as yet, it seems likely that the results obtained with carcinoma cells are also applicable to carcinomas of the lung.

ACKNOWLEDGMENTS

The in vivo observations were obtained in cooperation with Dr K.P. Dingemans of the Academical Medical Center of the University of Amsterdam. A large part of the results on adhesion molecules was obtained by Dr. O.P. Middelkoop who was supported by KWF-Netherlands Cancer Foundation grant NKI 80-6. The work on T-cell hybridomas was done in cooperation with Dr. P. De Baetselier of the Free University of Brussels, Belgium. In addition, Drs G. La Riviere and M.J. Stukart made important contributions. Technical assistance was provided by P. Van Bavel & I.V. Van de Pavert. We thank N. Ong for preparing micrographs and G.G.H. Meijerink for secretarial assistance.

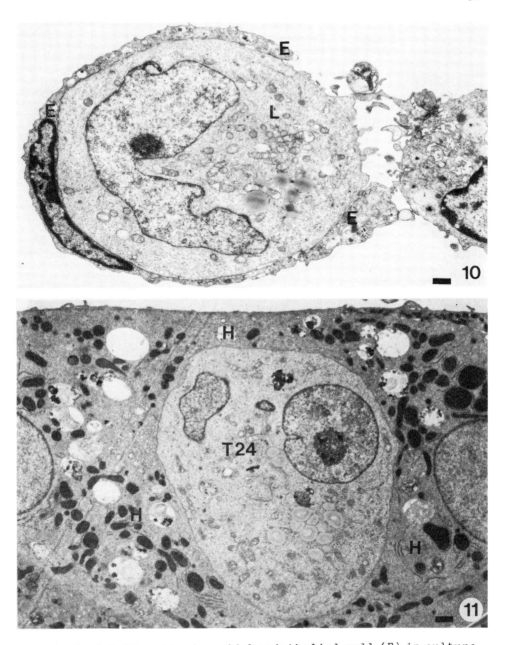

147

Fig. 10. Isolated hepatic sinusoidal endothelial cell (E) in culture adheres to and encircles a MB 6A lymphosarcoma cell (L). Encirclement was seen when a few percent rat serum was added. Bar: 1 um.

Fig. 11. Rat hepatocyte (H) culture to which T24 human bladder carcinoma cells had been added. After 24 h, several tumor cells had invaded, in much the same way as rat or mouse carcinoma cells. Bar: 1 um.

148

REFERENCES

1. Bross, I.D.J., Viadana, E. and Pickren, J. 1975. Do generalized metastases occur directly from the primary? J. Chron. Dis. 28, 149-159.
2. Roos, E., Dingemans, K.P., Van de Pavert, I.V., Van den Bergh Weerman, M. 1977. Invasion of lymphosarcoma cells into the perfused mouse liver. J. Natl. Cancer Inst. 58, 399-407.
3. Roos, E., Dingemans, K.P., Van de Pavert, I.V., Van den Bergh Weerman, M. 1978. Mammary carcinoma cells in mouse liver: Infiltration of liver tissue and interaction with Kupffer cells. Br. J. Cancer 38, 88-99.
4. Dingemans, K.P. 1973. Behaviour of intravenously injected lymphoma cells. A morphologic study. J. Natl. Cancer Inst. 51, 1883-1895.
5. Dingemans, K.P. 1974. Invasion of liver tissue by blood-borne mammary carcinoma cells. J. Natl. Cancer Inst. 53, 1813-1824.
6. Roos, E., Tulp, A., Middelkoop, O.P., Van de Pavert, I.V. 1984. Interactions between lymphoid tumor cells and isolated liver endothelial cells. J. Natl. Cancer Inst. 72, 1173-1180.
7. Roos, E., Van de Pavert, I.V., Middelkoop, O.P. 1981. Infiltration of tumour cells into cultures of isolated hepatocytes. J. Cell Sci. 47, 385-397.
8. Roos, E., Van de Pavert, I.V. 1982. Effect of tubulin-binding agents on the infiltration of tumour cells into primary hepatocyte cultures. J. Cell Sci. 55, 233-245.
9. Middelkoop, O.P., Roos, E., Van de Pavert, I.V. 1982. Infiltration of lymphosarcoma cells into hepatocyte cultures: inhibition by univalent antibodies against liver plasma membranes and lymphosarcoma cells. J. Cell Sci. 56, 461-470.
10. Roos, E., Middelkoop, O.P., Van de Pavert, I.V. 1984. Adhesion of tumor cells to hepatocytes: Different mechanisms for mammary carcinoma compared with lymphosarcoma cells. J. Natl. Cancer Inst. 73, 963-969.
11. Roos, E. 1984. Invasion of the liver by tumor cells. In: Liver Metastasis. Basic Aspects, Detection, Management. (C.J.H. Van der Velde & P.H. Sugarbaker, eds.), pp. 1-19. Martinus Nijhoff, The Hague.
12. Middelkoop, O.P., Van Bavel, P., Calafat, J. and Roos, E. 1985. Hepatocyte surface molecule involved in the adhesion of TA3 mammary carcinoma cells to rat hepatocyte cultures. Cancer Res. 45 (July 1985), in press.
13. Roos, E., Van de Pavert, I.V. 1983. Antigen-activated T-lymphocytes infiltrate hepatocyte cultures in a manner comparable to liver-colonizing lymphosarcoma cells. Clin. Exp. Metastasis 1, 173-180.
14. Roos, E., La Riviere, G., Collard, J.G., Stukart, M.J. and De Baetselier, P. Invasiveness and metastatic potential of T-cell hybridomas. Submitted for publication.
15. De Baetselier, P., Roos, E., Brys, L., Remels, L. & Feldman, M. 1984. Generation of an invasive and metastatic variant of a non-metastatic T-cell lymphoma by in vivo fusion with a normal host cell. Int. J. Cancer 34, 731-738.

APPLICATION OF MONOCLONAL ANTIBODIES IN IMAGING AND THERAPY

R.K.OLDHAM and M.H.WEST

1. INTRODUCTION

Surgery, radiotherapy and chemotherapy, the standard treatment modalities for cancer, have been in clinical medicine for more than two decades. The principles for the use of surgery and radiotherapy are very well established and mostly part of the standard practice of medicine. Chemotherapy is of more recent origin with a continued evolution in the use of chemotherapy with the advent of new drugs and new drug combinations over the past two decades. General principles are well established for the translation of toxic chemicals from the laboratory to the clinic.

In addition to surgical therapy, radiotherapy and chemotherapy there now exists a fourth modality of cancer treatment. This modality, biotherapy, uses biological substances and biological response modifiers as anticancer approaches (1). For biotherapy, many would simply apply principles established for the development of chemotherapy. Given the striking differences between biological substances and toxic chemicals, it may well be possible to bring biologicals through the process of development using different guidelines and principles then for drugs.

Biotherapy, in its modern form, is a very young modality. Certainly, biological substances have been used as medicinals for centuries. Most of these substances have been crude extracts, vaccines or other mixtures of biologically derived materials. The recent era of biotherapy began with the use of modern molecular biology to isolate, purify and produce large quantities of homogenous biological substances. Thus, highly purified biologicals have really only been available as medicinals over the past five years(2).

It is evident that antibody based biotherapeutic approaches offer the possibility for selective targeting of substances to tumor masses. There have been reports on the use of antibody alone with occasional clinical success(3). However, most of the clinical trials using unconjugated antibody have demonstrated targeting of the antibody to the tumor without clinical responses (4,5). Therefore, the selectivity of antibody will probably need to be exploited therapeutically in the form of an immunoconjugate using a drug, isotope or toxin.

Immunoconjugates with isotopes have received the most intensive clinical study thus far. There is strong evidence that tracer labeled monoclonal antibodies can be used to localize tumors in patients with melanoma, lymphoma, breast and gastrointestinal carcinomas(6,7). Very preliminary therapeutic trials in melanoma using more heavily labeled antibody preparations have also been reported(8). However, in contradiction to other immunoconjugates, isotopes have a certain "field effect". Differences among immunoconjugates are important considerations in the design of trials for toxin and drug based immunoconjugates compared to isotope based immunoconjugates.

Drugs are also undergoing early trials as toxic components of immunoconjugates. Toxins are not simply "strong drugs" as many toxin molecules are organic molecules of considerable size as compared to the smaller inorganic molecules from which most drugs have been derived. Of the 500,000 compounds which have been evaluated for use as chemotherapeutic agents, most have been eliminated because of high normal tissue toxicity. In effect, this means that many chemical substances have sufficient toxicity to be used as anticancer agents, but have excessive toxicity with respect to normal tissue damage. Thus, an immunoconjugate approach may allow a whole new therapeutic strategy using known toxic chemicals to be incorporated in an appropriate immunoconjugate as a selective targeting agent. While it may not be possible to select an antibody which has absolute specificity for the cancer cell, it is clear that many antibodies have some degree of selectivity for cancer cells as compared to normal cells. If this selectivity adds a level of selectivity to treatment then an immunoconjugate composed of antibody and drug may be an improvement over the unconjugated chemical.

A major advantage of antibody based biotherapeutic approaches is the ability to assess the tissue by appropriate immunohistochemical techniques and identify the antibody in the tissue. Immunoconjugates bearing isotopes can be directly detected by external scintigraphy. Antibodies bearing drugs or toxins molecules can be detected by immunohistochemistry. In the context of clinical trials evaluating immunotoxins, it will be necessary to biopsy cancerous deposits as well as selected normal tissues and look for the distribution of the immunotoxin in the tissues. Toxicity may well be predictable from lower dose trials by virtue of the selective localization in cancer tissues versus normal tissues. Unlike studies with chemicals, which are difficult to detect until toxicity becomes obvious, antibody based biotherapy gives one the opportunity to predict toxicity based on tissue

distribution. In fact, a combination approach may
someday be useful where isotope labeled immunotoxin
molecules are injected to allow calculation of tissue
distribution, predict toxicity and design clinical
trial strategies in a very sophisticated manner.

Current studies support the strategy of staging and
treating human malignancies with monoclonal antibodies
conjugated to isotopes, drugs and toxins. Several
reviews have been written on the use of monoclonal
antibody and heteroantisera in the treatment of cancer
(9-11). The purpose of this paper will be to provide
some perspective on the potential clinical use of
antibodies conjugated to drugs, isotopes and toxins.

2. DEVELOPMENT OF MONOCLONAL ANTIBODIES FOR THERAPY

A number of different murine monoclonal antibodies have
been assessed in clinical trials in patients with solid
tumors (9). More than ten antibodies for melanoma,
lung, breast and colon cancer have been described and
characterized. No doubt there will be a large variety
of new monoclonal antibodies of murine and human
derivation described in the future. Thus, it is
already apparent that the limitation for the use of
monoclonal antibodies as medicinals will not be a
shortage of antibodies.

Although the ideal antibody (i.e., absolute specificity
for cell surface antigens for a particular tumor) has
not been identified for human solid tumors, a number
have sufficient selectivity to warrant clinical
testing. Criteria to select monoclonal antibodies
appropriate for clinical trials will ultimately depend
on the projected role of the antibody in diagnosis or
treatment of the particular disease. Antibodies that
satisfy the criteria in Table 1 is more likely to have
clinical utility than those that do not, but it is
important to recognize that most of these judgements
are relative.

The antibody, whether conjugated or not, presumably
must reach the tumor bed to be effective. Smaller
antibodies (IgG rather than IgM) or antibody fragments
may be more likely to diffuse from the vascular
compartment out into the tumor bed. Our studies
indicate that the more whole IgG antibody infused into
the vascular compartment, the more antibody one
delivers to the tumor cell bed. We have even
demonstrated that doses of 200-500 mg of antibody can
saturate all sites on the tumor cells in cutaneous
malignant melanoma (4).

Table 1.

1. Antibody binds to a cell surface antigen;
2. Antibody binds with high affinity;
3. Antigen highly expressed on cell surface and found on most or (preferably) all cells in a tumor;
4. Antigen expressed at very low levels on a very limited number of normal tissues and/or found only on occasional cells in normal tissues;
5. Antigen-antibody complexes internalize*;
6. Antibody mediates cellular killing**;
7. Biodistribution studies reveal negligible uptake of antibody by RES.*

* Important for some immunoconjugates (toxins and drugs).
** Most important for unconjugated antibody.
* Especially important for conjugates.

There are certain important principles in the design and execution of clinical trials using monoclonal antibodies (9). It is necessary to have an active and competent laboratory to monitor the fate and distribution of antibody in clinical trials. It is crucial to demonstrate that antibody reached the tumor cells and bound to antigen in vivo (3,4,5). Additional testing should include antibody distribution, antigen saturation, antibody pharmacokinetics, circulating antigen, immune complexes, antiglobulin and anti-idiotypic responses to murine antibody.

Our studies have focused on two antibodies to study their safety and localization in three different cancers.

Table 2. Monoclonal antibody protocols at the BRMP-NCI.

Antibody	Disease	Number of patients	Dose	Schedule	Length of infusion (hr)	Dose escalation*
T101	CLL	7	1,10,50	biweekly	2	fixed
T101	CLL	6	50,100	biweekly	50	fixed
T101	CTCL	8	1,10,50	biweekly	2,50	fixed
T101	CTCL	3	100,200,500	biweekly	2†	escalating
9.2.27	melanoma	13	1,10,50,100 200,500	biweekly	2	escalating
9.2.27	melanoma	7	100 mg x5, 500 mg‡	daily	2	fixed
Anti-idiotype	CLL	1	10,20,50,100 200,500	biweekly	4	escalating
^{111}In-T101	CTCL	10	1 mg T101 + 5 mCi ^{111}In§	once only	2-10	
^{111}In-9.2.27	melanoma	8	1 mg 9.2.27 + 5 mCi ^{111}In§	once only	2	

*Fixed: dose fixed for each patient with escalation between patients. Escalating: each patient receives multiple dose levels.
†Patients received 2 mg T101/hr for 4 hr to modulate the T65 antigen from circulating cells and then received a 6-hr infusion of high-dose T101 (100 mg, first week; 200 mg, second week; 500 mg, third week).
‡Patients received 5 daily doses of 100 mg of antibody, 4 weeks off therapy followed by a single infusion of antibody.
§Some patients received 10-50 mg of unlabeled T101 or 9.2.27 in addition to immunoconjugate.

A series of melanoma patients was treated with the 9.2.27 IgG/2a murine monoclonal antibody (4). This antibody recognizes a 250 kd glycoprotein/proteoglycan antigen on the surface of melanoma cells. It binds to 90% of melanomas freshly removed from patients, exhibits both high affinity and quantitatively high binding to melanomas, and does not appear to bind to normal tissues with the exception of occasional basal cells, blood vessels and sebaceous glands in the skin. For these reasons it appeared to be an excellent candidate antibody for early clinical trials. As shown in Table 3, antibody reaches tumor cells at doses above 10 mg, with a definite trend to greater staining with higher doses.

Table 3. In vitro* and in vivo[†] reactivity of 9.2.27 antibody with melanoma cells in cutaneous skin lesions.

| | | | 9.2.27 reactivity | | | |
| | | | Flow cytometry (%) % positive cells | | Immunoperoxidase[‡] score | |
Patient	Dose 9.2.27	Days Posttreatment	In vitro	In vivo	In vitro	In vivo
A.F.	Pretreatment	1	80	ND	++	-
	1 mg	1	92	0	++	-
D.F.	Pretreatment		83	ND	++	-
	1 mg	1	0	0	+	-
	50 mg	1	72	0	++	+
	200 mg	1	ND	ND	++	+
M.F.	Pretreatment		97	ND	++	+
	10 mg	1	98	2	+	-
	100 mg	1	72	50	+	+
	200 mg	4	98	91	+	+
B.C.	Pretreatment		90	ND	++	-
	200 mg	1	73	71	+	+
C.S.	Pretreatment		76	ND	++	-
	1 mg	1	91	0	++	-
	200 mg	1	41	35	++	+
A.T.	Pretreatment		0	ND	+	-
	50 mg	1	ND	ND	++	++
	200 mg	1	14	50	++	++
M.G.	Pretreatment		76	1	++	-
	50 mg	4	97	1	++	-
J.S.	Pretreatment		ND	ND	++	-
	50 mg	1	ND	ND	++	+
	100 mg	1	ND	ND	++	++

*In vitro reactivity refers to reactivity when excess 9.2.27 was added during the staining procedure.
[†]In vivo reactivity refers to enodogenously bound 9.2.27 after i.v. antibody therapy.
[‡]Staining of melanoma cells with 9.2.27 was graded on a + to ++ scale which represents a combination of both percent positive cells and intensity of staining.

At the 10 mg and 1 mg doses, we generally did not detect antibody in the tumor by these techniques. The flow cytometry studies indicated that, at 50-500 mg first binding to tumor cells and then saturation of all available binding sites on the tumors could be achieved. The latter finding is important for several reasons: (i) It defines the maximum useful dose for a single injection; (ii) It determines the dose range expected for immunoconjugate delivery; (iii) It ensures that maximum doses of immunoconjugate reach every cell decreasing the chances of selecting resistant cells due to suboptimal delivery; (iv) It insures that hypoxic cells, those farthest from blood vessel access, receive the maximum deliverable dose. The immunoperoxidase studies indicated that areas of tumor most accessible to blood vessels or lymphatic spaces stain first and only with higher doses (>100 mg) did the other cells bind detectable antibody.

Following these studies, it was next central to determine where else the antibody was going. Radioimmunolocalization using 9.2.27 conjugated to Indium-111 was done to study the biodistribution of the antibody. Labeled antibody does go to the reticuloendothelial system as well as to tumor. The hepatic uptake is especially significant, but studies with 131-I-labeled 9.2.27 by others have shown much less in that organ (0. Fodstad, personal communication), suggesting that it was the 111-In or the chelation method that accounted for much of the hepatic binding in our studies. These studies raise critical issues concerning the relevance of unlabeled antibody studies to conjugates since the effect of the conjugation procedure and the material conjugated may profoundly influence the biodistribution.

Phase I studies have also been performed with other antibodies to melanoma. Less extensive but confirmatory studies were done with antibody 48.7 directed at the same antigen recognized by 9.2.27 (5). Haughton and co-workers have reported clinical responses using an antiglycolipid (GD3) monoclonal antibody in patients with metastatic melanoma. Larson and co-workers have gone one step further and labeled antibodies to P97 with therapeutic doses of 131-I. Localization of the labeled antibody has been seen and evidence of minor tumor regression was noted (8). Thus, these early clinical trials have progressed rapidly from antibody alone to therapeutic attempts with labeled antibody. Recently, an antimelanoma antibody/toxin conjugate phase I clinical trial was initiated by Xoma Corporation. All of these studies, taken together, demonstrate the feasibility of the immunoconjugate approach and will no doubt lead to future trials that will begin to demonstrate efficacy (12,13).

Sears and co-workers treated more than 20 gastrointestinal cancer patients with antibody 17-1A (IgG2a) and demonstrated localization of the antibody in the tumor (3). From 15-1000 milligrams per patient have been given as single doses without severe side effects. Circulating immunoglobulin has been seen for as long as 50 days compared to 9.2.27 which has a half life of approximately 30 hours and disappears from the

serum within days and certainly by 1 week. This may be
due to the low affinity of 17-1A and its shedding from
the tumor cell surface. In addition, 17-1A has a much
wider normal tissue reactivity than 9.2.27 and thus the
"sink" for antibody deposition and subsequent shedding
is much larger.

Antiglobulin responses to   17-1A   appeared   to   be
dependent on the dose of antibody. Those patients
receiving doses above 366 milligrams showed   little
antimouse immunoglobulin responses whereas the patients
treated with lower   doses   developed   definite
antiglobulins. Sears reported   evidence   of clinical
antitumor responses in   at   least   three   of these
patients, and postulated that this salutory effect may
have been due   to   antibody-macrophage interactions
within the tumor   bed.   They   suggested   that   a
combination of high doses of antibody, to reduce the
antiglobulin response, and the use of an IgG2a subclass
might be a reasonable approach in studying further
patients using unconjugated   antibody   with
gastrointestinal carcinoma.

A study of recent serotherapy trials using monoclonal
antibody for solid tumors is shown in Table 5.

Table 4. Monoclonal antibody serotherapy trials in
          patients with   solid   tumors.

Institution	Disease	MoAB*
*U. of Penn. (Wistar)	GI** cancer	17-1A
UCLA	GI cancer	CCOLI
U.Cal.San Diego	Colon cancer	065
U.Cal.San Diego	Melanoma	Ab to p97 Ab to p240
Fred Hutchinson Cancer Center	Melanoma	Ab to p97
Swedish Hosp.Med. Center,Seattle	Melanoma	48.7 Ab to p97
National Cancer Institute	Melanoma	9.2.27
Sloan-Kettering, NYC	Melanoma	Anti-GD3

*Ab or antigen designation
**GI, gastrointestinal
These studies are referenced in (13).

From the published data some conclusions on monoclonal antibody therapy are tenable (9). The subclass of antibody, the affinity of the antibody, the presence or absence of circulating antigen and the antiglobulin response are all important factors in the clinical use of antibody preparations. For studies in patients with solid tumors, there are advantages to using smaller molecules (IgG vs IgM; antibody fragments vs whole antibody) in that the primary method of access from the vascular compartment to the tumor appears to be by passive diffusion across the endothelial surfaces.

Once the in vitro activity of the immunoconjugate is established, the next step is to utilize the human tumor xenograft system to assess in vivo activity. As is illustrated in Table 5, established, palpable human melanoma tumors can be growth inhibited or even regress with appropriate immunotoxin conjugates. In this particular system, it was interesting to note that the 9.2.27 gelonin immunotoxin was less effective than the ricin A chain immunoconjugate in vitro but was more effective in vivo. Obviously, the size of the conjugate, its stability and purity and the translation of the conjugate from the vascular compartment to the tumor site all can have significant effects on the antitumor activity of the immunoconjugate.

Table 5.   Treatment of Established Palpable Human Melanoma in   Nude Mice with 9.2.27   Gelonin

Days Post Inititation of Therapy	Treatment Group (mg tumor mass)		
	Control *	500 ugx1	500 ugx4
29	402±59	281±33	199±58**
49	1201±59	1260±140	556±64**

*. Tumor volumes upon initiation of treatment 84±8 mg. Values represent mean ± standard error of 6 animals per treatment group.

**. p <.05 versus control (Student's t-test)

Antigenic modulation and   internalization.   Antigen modulation may be of clinical importance due to the capacity of some tumors to   evade   the   potential effectiveness of unconjugated   monoclonal   antibody therapy by modulation of the target antigen (14,15). On the other hand, since antigen modulation is often accompanied by internalization of antigen-antibody complexes, as has been demonstrated for the T101 antibody (15) and for the J5 antibody to the common acute lymphoblastic leukemia antigen (CALLA) (16), modulation may serve as an efficient means of delivering toxins into tumor cells for therapeutic purposes.

In two solid tumor systems we have examined the role of modulation on the toxicity of conjugates. In these systems there was no correlation of modulation with the degree of conjugate cytoxicity. The most striking example of this was with gelonin and ricin A chain conjugated to the anti-melanoma antibody 9.2.27. Neither of these conjugates show detectable modulation of cell surface antigen, yet kill antigen-positive melanoma cells at 10^{-11} to 10^{-13} M (ID 50). In contrast to unconjugated 9.2.27, both ricin/A and gelonin conjugates were internalized to a high degree. Internalization, as measured by loss of trypsin sensitivity of cell bound antibody was analyzed on cultured melanoma cells. Thus, internalization was enhanced by conjugation with toxin yet without detectable modulation.

Conjugate potency and selectivity. Potency and selectivity in killing antigen-positive cells have been the most intensely studied aspects of toxin conjugates in vitro. Toxin conjugates have been reported to vary in potency from 10^{-7} to 10^{-12} M (ID50) (17,18). The most potent of these toxin conjugates have employed intact ricin (18) or abrin (19) rather than isolated A subunits, resulting in an increase in potency of 100 to 1000-fold. Intact toxins bind to cell surface carbohydrate through a site on the B chain, are internalized presumably through coated pits, and are released into the cytoplasm where the A chain binds to and inactivates the 60S subunit of ribosomes. Selectivity of intact toxin conjugates has been achieved through either incubation with galactose to inhibit B-chain binding to cell surface carbohydrate (20), covalent incorporation of galactose into the B chain (21), or binding of intact toxin to antibody in such a manner that the carbohydrate binding site of the B chain in sterically occluded (18). The percent of conjugate with exposed B chains in dependent on the type of toxin, as studied with ricin or abrin (19) and, in our hands, the antibody used for conjugation. A second potential drawback of whole toxin conjugates could be release of toxin from conjugate in vivo, leading to toxicity. Thus far, in our experience administration of intact abrin conjugates to guinea pigs and nude mice had little evident toxicity, indicating little release of whole toxin.

A major factor in conjugate potency and selectivity, which has not been well studied, is the antibody-antigen system used for conjugation. We have examined ricin/A and abrin/A, pokeweed antiviral protein (PAP) and gelonin, and whole abrin conjugates of 9.2.27 antibody to human melanoma and D3 antibody to guinea pig L10 hepatocellular carcinoma. All 9.2.27 conjugates were potent (10^{-14} M to 10^{-11} M ID50) and highly selective. However, D3 antibody formed potent conjugate only with intact abrin but not with any of the A chains or A chain-like toxins (PAP and gelonin). As an example, both D3 and 9.2.27 were conjugated to the same preparation of ricin/A. Although both conjugates were selective in killing antigen positive cells, the potency of the two conjugates are distinctly different. 9.2.27-ricin/A conjugate was 6000-fold more potent than D3-ricin/A against appropriate antigen-positive cells (5.5×10^{-13} M vs 3.3×10^{-9} M ID50). Our preliminary conclusion is that the potency of both sets of antibody conjugates correlate with the degree of internalization; 9.2.27 conjugates internalize up to 50% in 6 hr whereas only 10% of the D3-A/chain conjugate internalize over the same interval. Thus, both the type of toxin and the antibody used for conjugation are important in producing potent and selective conjugates.

The fate of antibody, once bound to tumor cells, is an important parameter for immunoconjugate studies. In contrast to antigens like CALLA and T65, which are antigens on lymphoid malignancies that undergo rapid modulation when bound by antibody, many antigens of solid tumors show little modulation. Even though there is no detectable modulation, there can be distinctions in the rate of in vivo turnover. The D3 antibody in L10 tumors shows a rapid accretion into tumor, with a maximum at 24 hr, with an equally rapid loss from tumor, similar to the rate of loss from normal organs. In contrast, the 9.2.27 antibody shows a slower rate of accretion in human melanoma, a steady state period for up to 5 days, then a gradual loss. These properties affect the quality of tumor imaging. The localization and turnover of antibody may also affect radiotherapy with alpha or beta emitting isotope conjugates, but may have little effect on the efficacy of toxin conjugates. Both antibodies, conjugated to toxins, have shown therapeutic effects against established palpable tumors (23,24)

3. RADIOIMMUNODETECTION OF TUMORS

The use of radioactive antibodies for tumor detection and localization began in the 1940's with 131 I labeled antibodies which were shown to localize in tissues to which antibody had been made (6). Antibodies to fibrin, gliomas, human chorionic gonadotrophin and carcinoembryonic antigen have all been labeled with iodine and other isotopes and used with varying success

to localize tumors. Radioiodinated antibodies have
also been prepared against alphafetoprotein, colon
antigens and prostatic acid phosphatase to localize
tumors producing these substances. In most cases,
these earlier studies used polyvalent antiserum and
iodinated antibodies. Localization of the
radioiodinated antibodies was seen but the sensitivity
of these tests was low and in most cases the antibodies
did not reveal tumors that could not be localized by
more conventional means. In addition, some
localization was seen in nontumorous tissues and very
complicated background subtraction methods were
sometimes used. A major problem early in these studies
was the localization of the antibodies in the
reticuloendothelial (RES) system.

More recent studies have utilized monoclonal antibodies
directed toward these same antigens often labeled with
131 I and sometimes using the 99 Tc or 111 Indium.
These studies have demonstrated that truly tumor
specific markers are not necessary for radioactive
antibodies to be useful in cancer detection. The
relative concentration of the antigen to which the
antibody is made must be greater in tumor compared to
normal tissues for such reagents to be useful. It is
also clear that radioimmunodetection and radiotherapy
are very different matters. Radioimmunodetection can
occur when some of the cells in the tumor are positive
for the antigen and when some of the antigen is located
outside the tumor. However, for radiotherapy there is
a much greater need for higher specificity to avoid
damage to other organs.

For radioimaging 9.2.27 was radiolabeled with 125 I and
assessed for radiolocalization in tumor and normal
tissues of normal and tumor-bearing animals. The 125I-
9.2.27 localized in vivo preferentially in 250K
antigen-expressing human melanomas (REMX-Met, SESX) but
not in low antigen-expressing tumors (LOX-L)
xenografted in nude mice. The imaging index of tumor
cells was positively correlated with the antigen
density of the various melanoma cell lines as measured
by flow cytometry. The nonspecific immunoglobulin P3
of the same IgG2a subclass as 9.2.27 did not localize
to xenografts of melanoma. The total amount of 125I-
9.2.27 accumulated in the tumor was directly
correleated with tumor size. However, the specific
radioactivity (cpm/g) in smaller tumors was higher than
that in larger tumors.

Nonspecific uptake and circulating antibody levels
differed between normals and tumor-bearers. The organs
of the reticuloendothelial system of normal mice
accumulated more labeled antibody than did those of
tumor-bearers, and conversely, tumor-bearers had higher

levels of circulating labeled antibody in the blood
than normals. The circulating labeled antibody in
tumor-bearers was still monomeric but had no detectable
antigen-binding capacity.

The 111 Indium-labeled murine monoclonal antibodies
(D3, 9.2.27) directed to tumor antigens of L10
hepatocarcinoma and human melanoma, respectively,
selectively localized antigen-positive target cells in
guinea pigs and nude mice. The fate of monoclonal
antibodies differed in the two antigen-antibody systems
after reacting with their corresponding tumor antigens
in vivo as reflected by patterns of distribution and
turnover in vivo. 9.2.27 continuously accumulated in
melanoma xenograft in nude mice after iv administration
with slow loss from tumor but more rapid loss from
normal tissues and thus demonstrated optimal imaging of
small tumors (about 5 mm) between 3 and 6 days after
injection of the radiolabeled antibody. In contrast,
D3 demonstrated a biphasic accumulation in the guinea
pig L10 hepatocarcinoma with a maximal activity on the
second day after administration and showed rapid loss
from both tumor and normal tissues. Nonspecific
accumulation of antibodies in liver and in kidney was
found both in syngeneic (nude mice) and xenogeneic
(guinea pig) hosts but was more pronounced in the
xenogeneic species. These results indicate that the
nature of the antigen-antibody interaction may be of
importance in selecting monoclonal antibodies for both
diagnosis and therapy of malignant diseases.

We have recently performed a series of studies using
the 9.2.27 antibody labeled with 111 Indium through
diethylenetriaminepentacetic acid (DTPA). With the use
of the 111 Indium conjugate, one; milligram of the
9.2.27 antibody with five millicures of label was
administered either alone or in combination with 50
milligrams of unconjugated antibody. Serum half life
of the labeled antibody alone was 3 hrs but when
injected with unconjugated antibody the labeled and
unlabeled antibody half life was approximately 30
hours. Masses as small as 0.5 x 0.5 cm were seen and
occult metastasis not detected by routine clinical
means were also detected. Unfortunately, there was
substantial uptake by the reticuloendothelial system
and it was clear that radioimmunodetection for heptatic
metastasis would not be feasible. 111 Indium has also
been chelated to T10 antibody which reacts with the T
15 antigen on T cells and radioimmunodetection studies
performed in patients with leukemia and lymphoma.
Visualization of involved nodes can easily be
accomplished using this technique, but again uptake by
the reticuloendothelial system is a limiting factor.
Studies are currently underway to determine how much
RES uptake is related to uptake of breakdown products.

Specificity was confirmed by the lack of uptake of 111
Indium labeled 9.2.27 in patients with cutaneous
lymphoma who imaged very well with 111 In labeled T101.
From our studies and those of others it is now clear
that radioimmunodetection of cancer is now a reality.
The best likelihood is that labeled antibodies will be
useful in staging patients with known progression and
in locating clinically silent lesions. There may soon
be a use for these methods in patients highly suspect
for a particular malignancy, but there is little hope
of using these reagents in the next 3-5 years for
screening or radioimmunodetection in normal populations.

REFERENCES

1. Oldham, R. K.: Biologicals and biological response
modifiers: the fourth modality of cancer treatment.
Cancer Treat. Rep. 68:221-232, 1984.

2. Oldham, R. D. and Smalley, R. V.: Immunotherapy:
The old and the new. J. Biol. Resp. Modif., 2:1-37,
1983.

3. Sears, H. F., Herlyn, D., Steplewski, A.,
Koprowski, H.: Effects of monoclonal antibody
immunotherapy on patients with gastrointestinal
adenocarcinomias. J. Biol. Resp. Modif. 3:138-150,
1984.

4. Oldham, R. K., Foon, K. A., Morgan, A. C.,
Woodhouse, C. S., Schroff, R. W., Abrams, P. G., Fer,
M., Schoenberger, C. S., Farrell, M., Kimball, E.,
Sherwin, S.A.: Monoclonal antibody therapy of
malignant melonoma: In vivo localization in cultaneous
metastasis after intravenous administration. J. Clin.
Onc. 2:1235-1242, 1984.

5. Goodman, G.D., Beaumier, P., Hellstrom, I.,
Fernybrough, B., Hellstrom, K.E.: Pilot trial of
murine monoclonal antibodies in patients with advanced
cancer. J. Clin. Onc. 3:340-352, 1985.

6. Goldenberg, D.M., DeLand, F.H.: History and status
of tumor imaging with radiolabeled antibodies. J.
Biol. Resp. Modif. 1:121-136, 1982.

7. Carrasquillo, J.D., Krohn, K.A., Beaumier, P. et
al: Diagnosis and therapy of solid tumors with
radiolabeled Fab. Cancer Treat. Rep. 68:317-328, 1984.

8. Larson, S.M., Carrasquillo, J.A., Keohn, K.A., et
al.: Localization of p97 specific Fab fragments in
human melanoma as a basis for radiotherapy. J. Clin.
Invest. 72:2101-2114, 1983.

162

9. Oldham, R. K., Monoclonal antibodies in cancer therapy. J. Clin. Onc, 1:582-590, 1983.

10. Foon, K.A., Bernhard, M., Oldham, R.K.: Monoclonal antibody therapy: assessment by animal tumor models. J. Biol. Resp. Modif., 1:277-304, 1982.

11. Dillman, R.: Monoclonal antibodies in the treatment of cancer. CRC Critical Reviews in Oncology/Hematology, 1:357-385, 1984.

12. Oldham, R.K.: Antibody-drug and antibody toxin conjugates, Rief A.E., Mitchell M.S. (Eds) Immunity to Cancer, Academic Press, New York. In press, 1985.

13. Oldham, R.K., Abrams, P.: Monoclonal antibody therapy of solid tumors. Martinus Nijhoff. In press, 1985.

14. Abrams, P.G., Morgan, A.C. Jr.,Schroff, R.W., Woodhouse, C.S., Carrasquillo, J., Stevenson, M.F. Fer, Oldham, R.K., Foon, K.A.: Monoclonal antibody studies in melanoma: In Monoclonal Antibodies and Cancer Therapy, Reisfield and Sell (Eds.) In press, 1984.

15. Schroff, R.W., Farrell, M.M., Klein, R.A., Oldham, R.K., Foon, K.A. T65 antigen modulation in a phase I monoclonal antibody trial with chronic lymphocytic leukemia patients. J. Immunol., 133:1641-1648, 1984.

16. Ritz, J., Pesando, J.M., Sallan, S.E., Clavell, L.A., Notis-McConarty, J., Rosenthal, P., Schlossman, S.F. 1981. Sero-therapy of acute lymphoblastic leukemia with monoclonal antibody. Blood 58:141.

17. Davis, M.-T.B., Preston, J.F. 1981. A conjugate of a amanitin and monoclonal immunoglobulin G to THY 1.2 antigen is selectively toxic to T lymphoma cells. Science 213:1385-1387.

18. Thorpe, P.E., Ross, W.C., Brown, A.N., Myers, C.D., Cumber, A.J., Foxwell, B.M., Forrester, J.T. 1984. Blockade of the galactose-binding sites of ricin by its linkage to antibody. Specific cytotoxic effects of the conjugates. Eur. J. Biochem. 140:63-71.

19. Godal, A., Funderud, S., Fodstad, O., Pihl, A. 1984. Comparison of abrin and ricin immunotoxins. In: Protides of the Biological Fluids, XXXII Annual Colloquium. H. Peeters, (Ed.) Elsevier, Amsterdam, Vol. 32, 1984.

20. Callera, D.A., Youle, R.J., Neville, D.M., Kersey, J.H. 1982. Bone marrow transplantation across major histocompatibility barriers. V. Protection of mice from lethal GVHD by pretreatment of donor cells with monoclonal anti Thy 1.2 coupled to the toxic lectin ricin. J. Exp. Med. 155:949.

21. Houston, L.L. 1983. Inactivation of ricin using 4 azidophenyl-beta-D galacto pyranoside and 4 diazophenyl-beta-D galacto pyranoside. J. Biol. Chem. 258:7208-7212.

22. Weinstein, J.N., Steller, M.A., Kennan, A.M., Covell, D.G., Key, M.E., Sieber, S.M., Oldham, R.K., Hwang, K.M., Parker, R.J. 1983. Monoclonal antibodies in the lymphatics: Selective delivery. Science 222:423-426.

23. Morgan, A.C. Jr., Pavanasasivam, G., Hwang, K.M., Woodhouse, C.S., Schroff, R.W., Foon, K.A., Oldham, R.K. 1984. Preclinical and clinical evaluation of a monoclonal antibody to a human melanoma associated antigen. In: Protides of the Biological Fluids, XXXII Annual Colloquium. H. Peeters, (Ed.) Elsevier, Amsterdam, 32:773-777, 1985.

24. Hwang, K. M., Foon, K.A., Cheung, P.H., Pearson, J.W., Oldham,, R.K. 1984. Selective antitumor effect of a potent immunoconjugate composed of the A chain of abrin and a monoclonal antibody to a hepatoma-associated antigen. Cancer Res., 44:4578-4586, 1984.

CURRENT CONCEPTS IN THE THERAPY OF SMALL CELL LUNG CANCER

L.AUSTIN DOYLE and JOSEPH AISNER

Small cell lung cancer (SCLC) is a highly malignant neoplasm
afflicting between 25,000 and 30,000 persons each year in the
United States (1). SCLC is clinically differentiated from other
types of lung cancer by rapid growth, early metastases and both
chemo- and radiosensitivity (2). Before 1970, patients with SCLC
were treated with surgical resection of the tumor or chest
irradiation. In the early 1970's it became apparent that SCLC was
a disseminated disease in the vast majority of SCLC patients, even
among those whose tumor was clinically confined to the chest at
the time of diagnosis (3). With careful staging, about one third
of patients have such clinically limited disease. The realization
of the disseminated nature of this disease led to the application
of chemotherapy which, when added to chest irradiation, was
superior to radiation alone in the treatment of localized disease
(4). Initial chemotherapy trials consisted of single agents, but
it soon became apparent that combinations of 3 to 4 drugs had a
greater impact on response and survival leading to a small
percentage of cures (5). Using modern chemotherapy, radiotherapy
and supportive care, the three year disease-free survival is still
only 8-10 percent overall and problems of late tumor recurrence,
second malignancy and treatment toxicity can affect survival in
these long-term survivors (6). In order to understand the current
treatment approach, it is appropriate to consider the impact of
various therapeutic strategies over the past decade and to
consider new information on the biology of SCLC that may be used
to improve the diagnosis and therapy of this disease.

1. CHEMOTHERAPY

Early in the drug therapy history of SCLC, many agents were shown
to have antitumor activity but few new active agents have been
discovered since 1976. Complicating the identification of new
agents is the development of pleiotropic drug resistance during

initial therapy with "standard" agents. SCLC patients entered on
recent phase II trials of new agents have usually failed 3 to 6
active drugs as well as radiation therapy. They also often have
poor performance status and a heavy tumor burden. As an example
of this phenomenoma etoposide (VP16) had a response rate of 45% in
untreated SCLC, but less than 10% in patients who relapsed after
combination chemotherapy (7).

Considering the number of active agents there are many possible
combinations but most active combinations in the treatment of SCLC
include such active single agents as vincristine,
cyclophosphamide, doxorubicin (adriamycin), etoposide (VP16), CCNU
and methotrexate. Among the most active combinations are: 1)
cyclophosphamide, doxorubicin and etoposide, 2) vincristine,
cyclophosphamide and doxorubicin; and 3) cyclophosphamide, CCNU
and vincristine with either methotrexate or etoposide.

When optimally given, these regimens will result in a response
frequency greater than 80% for both limited and extensive stage
SCLC. Combination chemotherapy produces complete responses (CRs)
in 40-65% of patients with limited disease and 15-40% of patients
with extensive disease. This is variable between series and
depends on staging and restaging. The survival are however more
uniform in results. The median survival data for patients with
limited SCLC is greater than 14 months and greater than 8 months
for those with extensive disease (5). The group of patients which
achieves CR has a significantly longer survival than those who
achieve only a partial response (PR) and only patients who achieve
CR have the potential for long term survival. "Optimal"
chemotherapy is therefore predicated upon maximizing the
percentage of patients achieving a CR by administering maximally
tolerated doses which in turn may have significant hematologic
toxicity.

One prospectively randomized trial specifically addressed the
question of increasing drug dosage. Cohen et al. (8) compared the
results of cyclophosphamide, methotrexate and CCNU in standard
outpatient doses with those achieved by doubling the doses of

these agents and administering them in an inpatient setting. The
overall response rate and median survival were markedly improved
in the high-dose chemotherapy group. CRs and disease-free
survival at two years were noted only with the more intensive
regimen.

With such a dose response demonstrated in SCLC, numerous studies
were undertaken to determine if even more intensive therapy were
better still (9,10,11). Some studies added locoregional
irradiation or autologous bone marrow "rescue" to the intensive
induction therapy (12,13) or as consolidation (14). In the latter
case, a critical step was to verify that the marrow was free of
metastatic disease through the use of techniques such as
cytofluorography or agarose cloning (15,16). Some intensive
regimens were tested in poor-risk groups such as patients with
extensive disease or those who had relapsed from initial induction
therapy (17,18). While most of these studies of intensive
induction therapy were not randomized between intensive and
standard therapy, the more intensive regimens appear to produce
higher response rates. However, none of these approaches seem to
have produced a major improvement in survival, especially in
extensive SCLC, in part because the advantage is offset by an
increased induction mortality. There thus appears to be a limit
beyond which higher dosage escalations appear to produce only
increased toxicity without substantially increased therapeutic
benefit. Similarly, late intensification regimens, designed to
intensively attack a small residual tumor burden, do not appear to
have improved survival in SCLC and have been discontinued in most
centers.

During successful therapy of SCLC, tumor regression tends to occur
quickly and in some reports the CRs occur within the first two
induction cycles (19). However, in other reports CRs can occur
with the fifth or sixth cycle. This has led to some confusion
concerning the duration of chemotherapy. Since most CRs in SCLC
eventually relapse, one common approach is to continue
chemotherapy until relapse occurs or 24 months as an arbitrary cut
off. Several recent studies reported on SCLC treatment using only

six cycles of combination chemotherapy along with chest
irradiation (20,21,22). While these studies were not randomized
against a maintenance arm, the results of shorter duration
treatment appear similar to those achieved by continuing therapy
for more prolonged periods. There is very little information
which has tested this issue, however. The CALGB conducted a trial
in which SCLC patients who achieved a CR were randomized to
receive either maintenance therapy with the induction regimen
given every other month or to no maintenance therapy (23).
Thirty-six patients with limited disease achieved a CR. The CR
duration of 4.0 months for the maintainence versus 3.5 months for
the non-maintenance therapy group was not significantly
different. The group that received maintenance therapy, however,
had a significantly longer survival than the unmaintained group
(16.8 versus 6.8 months, p=0.01). Therefore, some patients can
achieve longterm disease free survival with relatively short
durations of chemotherapy, especially when concurrent chest
radiation therapy is added. However, the length of maintenance
therapy needed to maximize survival for all complete responders is
still undetermined. Patients who achieve less than a CR have a
very short survival and in general should be maintained on
chemotherapy until the time of disease progression. One potential
approach to these patients is to test new agents in patients with
PRs.

Early studies in SCLC showed that some tumors which progressed
during combination chemotherapy occasionally responded to a second
combination, suggesting the possible use of multiple
combinations. Goldie and Coldman (24) proposed that tumors
continually mutate toward drug resistance and that, where all
drugs can not be combined, alternating several chemotherapy
combinations during initial therapy might prevent the development
of drug resistance. The NCI-VA group reported results with
alternating CMC (cyclophosphamide, methotrexate and CCNU) and VAP
(vincristine, doxorubicin and procarbazine) (25). These
combinations were considered to be non-cross resistant because
some patients whose disease progressed during CMC responded
following VAP. While an improved CR rate was seen in patients

receiving the alternating combinations, survival was not
significantly altered. Another randomized study was reported by
Aisner et al. (26). One hundred and nine patients were randomized
to receive either ACE (doxorubicin, cyclophosphamide, etoposide)
or ACE alternating with a non-cross resistant combination of COMP
(CCNU, vincristine, methotrexate and procarbazine). There were no
significant differences in the results achieved by the two
regimens in terms of response rate, response duration or
survival. Analysis of more than 30 studies using "alternating
non-cross resistant combinations" indicates that this strategy
offers no major advantage over the intensive use of one regimen
until disease progression followed by therapy with another
chemotherapy combination. Regardless of the conclusions of the
authors, most of whom were negative to this approach, none of
these studies achieved better survival than so called "state of
the art" 15 month and 8 month median survivals for limited and
extensive disease respectively or greater percentage of long term
survival (27).

Clinical trials in SCLC based on maximizing tumor cell kill by
alterations in drug scheduling are still in their infancy but this
approach has already yielded some provocative results. Flow
cytometry techniques have demonstrated that sequential changes
occur in the distribution of tumor cells in the different phases
of the cell cycle following chemotherapy (28,29). Based on this,
drug combinations are being designed to take advantage of the
cell-cycle changes induced by the initial therapy. For example
Osterlind et al. (30) reported on a randomized trial of 254 SCLC
patients in which some patients received etoposide on a schedule
according to cell kinetic information. The objective was to
administer etoposide at a time when the most cells were in the S
phase of the cell cycle. In this study, patients who received
drug based on kinetic data had a prolonged survival compared to
the other group receiving the same drugs on a different
schedule. This raises the possibility of multiple permutations
and the potential use of additional cell cycling agents.

2. RADIATION THERAPY IN COMBINATION WITH CHEMOTHERAPY

Small cell lung cancer is the most radiosensitive form of lung
cancer, but the specific role of radiotherapy in the treatment of
this disease is still being defined. Two-thirds of patients who
achieved a CR on chemotherapy alone will relapse with systemic
disease although one half of this group (one third of all CR's)
will also have relapsed intrathoracic disease. The other third of
patients will have only intrathoracic relapses. Thus two thirds
of patients will, in addition to other sites, relapse in areas of
prior disease. This pattern of relapse also holds for patients
with extensive disease (31). Radiotherapy cannot control systemic
disease, but its application may alter the local failure rate.
Recent trials of combined modality treatment have examined relapse
patterns after chest irradiation in patients with limited SCLC.
Combined modality therapy leads to a lower rate of intrathoracic
relapses though this rate still approaches 33% (31,32). More
controversial is whether combined modality treatment increases the
time to initial recurrence or changes the survival outcome. The
toxicity of combined modality therapy is higher than chemotherapy
alone, especially with pulmonary, hematologic and esophageal
morbidity. The CR rate in limited SCLC appears to be higher with
combined modality therapy, but many features are obliterated by
the postradiation scarring. Furthermore in most studies survival
with combined modality is not greater than with chemotherapy
alone. While trials of sequential chemotherapy and radiotherapy
(sandwich technique) have never shown a survival advantage to
combined modality therapy for limited SCLC, several recent
randomized trials of concurrent chemotherapy and radiotherapy
suggest superior results in the percentage of two year disease-
free survivors and a trend toward increased overall survival in
the arms containing radiotherapy (33,34,35,36). One of these
studies, conducted at the National Cancer Institute, showed the
importance of careful planning of the radiation fields in
minimizing the toxicity of combined modality treatment. Custom-
shaped blocks were designed as would be done in mantle irradiation
for Hodgkin's disease. Since SCLC often responds rapidly to
concurrent chemo- and radiotherapy, a "shrinking field" technique

was used. A new radiograph for planning treatment was taken each week and, if significant reduction in tumor bulk occurred, new blocks were fashioned to spare lung toxicity. While such meticulous attention to detail would be difficult to duplicate generally, the preliminary results indicate that advances in treatment planning, such as the use of CT scanning may succeed in improving survival in these patients. However, for all the current studies of concurrent combined modality studies, the addition of chest irradiation, for loco-regional disease, to currently available moderately intense chemotherapy adds a consistant but only modest benefit to either the median survival or disease free survival over chemotherapy alone. Only one study combined maximally aggressive chemotherapy with concurrent irradiation and in this study the toxicity appeared prohibitive (37). It remains to be tested if such an approach would be feasible on a wider scale.

The other potential indication of radiotherapy in SCLC is for "prophylactic" brain irradiation in an attempt to reduce the incidence of relapses in the CNS. Brain metastases are clinically detected in approximately 15% of SCLC patients at the time of diagnosis and develop clinically in an additional 20% of patients during the natural course of the disease (38,39,40). In addition, as modern chemotherapy regimens have led to improved survival for SCLC patients, the frequency of brain metastases has increased with the duration of survival (41,42). Thus precisely those patients who derive the greatest benefit from treatment of their disease are those at the greatest risk of suffering this complication.

Retrospective studies in over 1300 patients with SCLC indicates that the incidence of relapse in the brain can be reduced from 22 to 8% by prophylactic cranial irradiation (PCI) (43). This conclusion has been confirmed in subsequent randomized trials in radiotherapy doses from 24 Gy to 30 Gy (44,45). There is no overall improvement in survival of SCLC patients treated with PCI, although the subgroup of patients who achieved a CR has shown an increased fraction of long-term disease-free survivors. One explanation for the lack of significant survival advantage is that the numbers of patients needed to show a significant benefit for PCI (25% of 30%) is prohibitive to any trial. At the UMCC a prospectively randomized trial and a review of our entire PCI experience demonstrated a highly significant delay to the onset of brain metastases among individuals receiving PCI compared to those not receiving PCI (46). PCI virtually eliminated the CNS as a primary site of failure. At the NCI-Navy, Rosen et al. found the actuarial fraction of complete responders alive at 30 months was 32 and 14% in patients who did and did not receive PCI respectively (47). Only in complete responders to systemic treatment might PCI be expected to have any impact on survival since patients with partial or no response die rapidly from uncontrolled systemic disease. Since the timing of PCI does not appear to be critical, the PCI can be given with maximal impact after induction chemotherapy to those patients who have achieved CR.

3. TREATMENT AFTER RELAPSE

The results of therapy are poor for patients who relapse with SCLC and the median survival from relapse is short, often only 7-8 weeks (48). Since single agent treatment after SCLC relapse has been discouraging, several groups have tried to identify combinations of active drugs that may be useful to patients after initial therapy has failed. Poplin et al. (49) reported on CCNU, vincristine, methotrexate and procarbazine for patients who relapsed on cyclophosphamide, doxorubicin and etoposide. Seventeen percent of the patients obtained a CR in this study but these were the better performance status, limited disease group. Cohen et al. (50) used vincristine, doxorubicin and procarbazine following therapy with cyclophosphamide, methotrexate and CCNU and reported a 24% CR rate. Recently, several groups have reported over 50% total response rates in relapsed SCLC patients treated with the combination of etoposide and cisplatin (51,52). While results with cisplatin alone in SCLC are conflicting, with reported response rates from 6-31 percent, there is both experimental and clinical evidence for true synergy between cisplatin and etoposide. The results of secondary treatment

studies suggest a particular benefit for patients who relapse from
chemotherapy in the chest alone and these patients may be candi-
dates for newer combined modality studies. At the UMCC we are
studying hypofractionated chest irradiation and combination
chemotherapy. Patients who relapse with specific symptoms should
undergo irradiation to that site if this modality were not
previously employed.

Most patients who survive disease free beyond 2 years will be long
term survivors, but occasionally patients will relapse late, and
therapy at this point is uncertain. Patients who relapse late
(beyond 24 months) after induction therapy may have a better
response rate to further chemotherapy than patients who relapse
early, however. A report from the NCI described six patients with
SCLC who relapsed more than 24 months after the induction of a CR
(53). Three of the six patients had responses lasting 9+ to 18
months, after reinduction with most or all of the drugs used
initially. This finding may indicate that the drug resistance
seen in SCLC tumors may be genetically unstable or that these
patients are susceptible to new SCLC tumors.

4. LONG-TERM SURVIVORS OF SCLC

Over the past decade, information has accumulated on the
characteristics of patients who are long-term survivors (LTS) of
SCLC. Matthews et al. (54) reported on 121 patients, collected
from various studies, including some older studies, who lived for
more than two years after the initiation of therapy. Based on
this review, one could project that at least 7% of all patients
with SCLC will be LTS. In these series 13% of the patients had
limited disease and 2% had extensive disease. Since treatment has
improved slightly and will likely continue to improve, these
figures should be base values.

Some patients alive and disease-free two years after starting
treatment for SCLC will relapse with SCLC or succumb to other
tumors (55). Among the possible other tumors, non-small cell lung
cancers(NSCLC) have been the most frequently seen. In about 5% of

SCLC cases a mixed SCLC/NSCLC tumor is discovered at initial
biopsy (56). At necropsy, nearly 30% of such mixed tumors are
noted (57). In patients successfully treated for SCLC who relapse
late with NSCLC, it is conceivable that a slower-growing and drug-
resistant histology might predominate. This is highly plausable
since both tumors have similar epidemiologic contributing factors
such as cigarette smoking. Alternatively, a second lung primary
tumor may develop under the influence of chemotherapy. Second
tumors of other organs, including acute leukemia, also have been
recorded in the LTS group.

A recent report by Johnson et al. (58) described a late occurring
CNS syndrome among SCLC patients especially those who received
PCI. Nine of eleven long-term survivors had significant
abnormalities by psychological testing including memory loss and
impaired intellectual testing. Head CT scans in 4/10 patients
showed cerebral atrophy. Five of 14 total patients were severely
incapacitated by the CNS syndrome. Many other investigators are
currently evaluating their data to determine incidence,
contributing factors, treatments, etc. to help assess this CNS
syndrome and whether there is any specific drug-radiation
interaction.

5. NEW APPROACHES IN SCLC THERAPY

One potentially important modality in the treatment of SCLC is the
use of anticoagulants. The coagulation process may have an
important role in the formation of metastases. Thus,
anticoagulation may reduce metastases, increase drug penetration
into small vessels or act in some other unexplained manner.
Regardless of mechanism, there are several hints which suggest a
role for anticoagulation in the treatment of SCLC. One study
randomized patients to receive combination chemotherapy with or
without Warfarin (59). The median survival in the group treated
with Warfarin was twice that of the chemotherapy alone group and
the Warfarin-treated group also had a significant increase in the
time to disease progression. In a following study the CALGB
tested anticoagulation in extensive disease using Warfarin with
combination chemotherapy. The preliminary results (60) confirm

the findings of the Veterans Hospital studies and a more
aggressive limited disease study is currently underway by the
CALGB.

At a recent meeting of the International Association for the Study
of Lung Cancer at Gleneagles, Scotland, the pathology panel
collapsed some of the SCLC subtyping because they found no significant clinical differences between small cell carcinoma of the
oat-cell type and of the intermediate-cell subtype a* (polygonal
or fusiform cells) (61). These are now all called "small cell."
Clinical studies of intermediate-cell subtype b*, which contains
an admixture of large cells with prominent nucleoli, (now called
small cell/large cell) indicate that these tumors are associated
with more virulent growth, relative resistance to chemotherapy and
radiotherapy and shorter survival times than "pure" small-cell
carcinomas. Cultures of small-cell carcinomas show classic,
variant and multipotent cell lines. The variant lines look like
large cells and have a higher growth rate and cloning efficiency
than classic SCLC (62). While the variant cell lines have the
SCLC markers of creatine-kinase-BB, neuron-specific enolase and
the 3p chromosomal deletion, they have lost bombesin and dopa
decarboxylase production and show amplification of the c-myc
oncogene (63). In vitro studies show that the variant cell lines
have greater resistance to chemotherapy and radiotherapy,
resembling the small cell/large cell grouping (64). Multipotent
cell lines may grow squamous or adenocarcinoma cells or both and
constitute evidence for a unitarian origin for all bronchial
carcinomas.

An enormous amount of information has recently been acquired on the
biology of SCLC which clearly distinguishes SCLC cells from NSCLC
cells (65). Permanent lines of SCLC cells can now be established
from patients with a high degree of efficiency using a defined
serum-free medium containing specific growth factors (66). These
"clonable" cell lines retain many of the biochemical properties of
the patient's tumor despite years of passage in cell culture.
When inoculated into nude mice, these cells form tumors with
typical SCLC histology. SCLC cells are distinguished from other

lung cancer cells by morphology, by a deletion of the short arm of the third chromosome (67) and by production of factors, which link them to APUD tumors, such as bombesin, dopa decarboxylase, neuron specific enolase and the BB isoenzyme of creatine kinase (68). Studies with two-dimensional gel electrophoresis of SCLC and NSCLC cells have revealed distinct surface protein phenotypes characteristic of these tumors (69). The anti-Leu 7 monoclonal antibody reacts against SCLC but not NSCLC cells (70).

Cultured SCLC cell lines may be used as models to: 1) test new drugs or synergistic drug pairs, 2) select new modalities of therapy and 3) explore mechanisms of drug resistance (71,72). It may yet be possible to develop screening panels of cell lines to assess potential new drugs. Furthermore, these methods may help to reclassify tumors and change therapy for one or more subgroups of patients.

Several of the characteristic proteins produced by SCLC cells may have potential as clinical markers for following SCLC. Carney and coworkers (73) found that serum neuron-specific enolase (NSE) was elevated in 69% of 94 patients with SCLC at the time of diagnosis, especially in patients with extensive disease. Serial measurements of NSE in patients receiving combination chemotherapy showed an excellent correlation between serum NSE and clinical response. Serum NSE levels generally normalized in the case of complete remission and rose again with relapse, with the rise sometimes predating clinical relapse by several months.

Some peptide hormones produced by SCLC cells, which cause para-neoplastic syndrome in the patient, may have auto-stimulatory effects upon the tumor cells themselves. Two hormones, arginine vasopressin and bombesin, are known to be produced by SCLC cells, which have receptors for these hormones and which are stimulated to proliferate in vitro by nanomolar quantities of these hormones. These auto-stimulatory mechanisms may potentially be blocked by immunologic means. For example, Cuttitta and coworkers (74) have produced a monoclonal antibody that binds to the C-terminal region of bombesin and prevents the binding of the hormone to its receptor. This antibody inhibits the clonal growth of SCLC cells in vitro and can cure nude mice bearing established SCLC tumors. In addition, this antibody has been successfully used to distinguish SCLC cells in immunohistochemical tissue staining and to localize tumors implanted in nude mice by scanning when labelled with a radionuclide. This has obvious important implications for staging.

SCLC cells have been recently found to have markedly decreased expression of the class I major histocompatibility complex (MHC) antigens HLA-A,B,C and beta-2 microglobulin (B_2m). The deficit appears to be caused by decreased mRNA transcription of these species (75). The absence of class I MHC antigens may enable SCLC cells to escape immunologic surveillance and may partially explain the early metastases and rapid local growth of SCLC compared to NSCLC tumors which have abundant expression of these antigens. The deficit in HLA-A,B,C and B_2m expression can be largely reversed by treatment with interferon either in vitro or in patients (76). While the response rate in established SCLC treated with interferon is not encouraging (77), one recent report indicates that interferon may decrease the rate of proliferation in SCLC and may have a radiosensitizing effect (78). One potential application of this approach, however, would be to use interferon after chemotherapy debulking.

6. CONCLUSION

Current clinical results show that SCLC is a highly treatable and potentially curable neoplasm. The demonstration of a group of long-term disease free survivors has stimulated a huge research effort in the biology of this disease. These studies appear to be producing results with the potential to impact on the survival of SCLC patients. SCLC cell lines should allow the identification of new active chemotherapeutic agents and permit biochemical analysis of the drug resistance seen with older agents. The development of new treatment modalities based on advances in tumor cell biology may allow most patients to realize the long-term survival benefit currently seen in only a few.

REFERENCES

1. Cancer Statistics. 1980; CA13-28.

2. Cohen MH, Matthews MT: Small cell bronchogenic carcinoma: a distinct clinicopathologic entity. Sem Oncol 1978; 5:234

3. Bleehen NM, Bunn PA, Cox JD, et al.: Role of radiation therapy in small cell anaplastic carcinoma of the lung. Cancer Treat Rep 1983; 67:11

4. Bergsagel DC, Jenkin RDT, Pringle JF, et al.: Lung cancer: Clinical trial of radiotherapy alone vs. radiotherapy plus cyclophosphamide. Cancer 1972; 30:621

5. Aisner J, Alberto P, Bitran J, et al.: Role of chemotherapy in small cell lung cancer: A consensus report of the International Association for the Study of Lung Cancer Workshop. Cancer Treat Rep 1983; 67:37.

6. Hansen HH, Rorth M, Aisner J: Management of small cell carcinoma of the lung. In: Contemporary Issues in Clinical Oncology: Lung Cancer, Aisner J (ed), New York, Churchill Livingstone, 1985, pp. 269

7. Broder LE, Cohen MH, Selawry OS: Treatment of bronchogenic carcinoma II: small cell. Cancer Treat Rev 1977; 4:219.

8. Cohen MH, Craven PJ, Fossieck BE, et al.: Intensive chemotherapy of small cell bronchogenic carcinoma. Cancer Treat Rep 1977; 61:349

9. Brower M, Ihde DC, Johnston-Early A, et al.: Treatment of extensive stage small cell bronchogenic carcinoma: effects of variation in intensity of induction chemotherapy. Am J Med 1983; 75:993

10. Farha P, Spitzer G, Valdivieso M, et al.: Treatment of small cell bronchogenic carcinoma (SCBC) with high dose chemotherapy (CT) and autologous bone marrow transplantation (ABMT). Proc Am Soc Clin Oncol 1981; 22:496.

11. Aisner J, Whitacre M, Van Echo DA, et al.: Doxorubicin, cyclophosphamide and VP16-213 (ACE) in the treatment of small cell lung cancer. Cancer Chemother Pharmacol 1982; 7:187.

12. Spitzer G, Dicke KA, Litam J, et al.: High-dose combination chemotherapy with autologous bone marrow transplantation in adult solid tumors. Cancer 1980; 45:307

13. Souhami RL, Harper PG, Linch D, etal.: High-dose cyclophosphamide with autologous marrow transplantation as initial treatment of small cell carcinoma of the bronchus. Cancer Chemother Pharmacol 1982; 8:31

14. Klastersky J, et al. and the EORTC Lung Cancer Working Party: Cisplatin, adriamycin and etoposide (CAV) for remission induction of small cell bronchogenic carcinoma. Evaluation of efficacy and toxicity and pilot study of a "late intensification" with autologous bone-marrow rescue. Cancer 1982; 50:652

15. Carney D, Broder L, Edelstein M, et al.: Experimental studies of the biology of human small cell lung cancer. Cancer Treat Rep 1983; 67:27.

16. Vindelov LL, Hansen HH, Christensen IJ, et al.: Clonal heterogeneity of small-cell anaplastic carcinoma of the lung demonstrated by flow-cytometric DNA analysis. Cancer Res 1980; 40:4295.

17. Abeloff MD, Ettinger DS, Order SE, et al.: Intensive induction chemotherapy in 54 patients with small cell carcinoma of the lung. Cancer Treat Rep 1981; 65:639

18. Hande KR, Oldham RK, Fer MF, et al.: Randomized study of high-dose versus low-dose methotrexate in the treatment of extensive small cell lung cancer. Am J Med 1982; 73:413

19. Morstyn G, Ihde DC, Lichter AS, et al.: Small cell lung cancer 1973-1983: Early progress and recent obstacles. Int J Rad Oncol Biol Phys 1984; 10:515

20. Byhardt RW, Cox JD, Holoye PY, Libnoch JA: The role of consolidation irradiation in combined modality therapy of small cell carcinoma of the lung. Int J Radiat Oncol Biol Phys 1979; 5:2043

21. Feld R, Evans WK, Yeoh JL, et al.: Combined modality induction therapy without maintenance chemotherapy for small cell carcinoma of the lung (SCCL). Proc Am Soc Clin Oncol 1981; 22:494.

22. Holoye PY, Libnoch JA, Byhardt RW, Cox JD: Integration of chemotherapy and radiation therapy for small cell carcinoma of the lung. Int J Radiat Oncol Biol Phys 1982; 8:1593

23. Maurer LH, Tulloh M, Weiss RB, et al.: A randomized combined modality trial in small cell carcinoma of the lung. Comparison of combination chemotherapy-radiation therapy versus cyclophosphamide-radiation therapy. Effects of maintenance chemotherapy and prophylactic whole brain irradiation. Cancer 1980; 45:30

24. Goldie JH, Coldman AJ, Gudauskas GA: Rationale for the use of alternating non-cross-resistant chemotherapy. Cancer Treat Rep 1982; 66:439

25. Cohen MH, Ihde DC, Bunn PA jr, et al.: Cyclic alternating combination chemotherapy for small cell bronchogenic carcinoma. Cancer Treat Rep 1979; 63:163

26. Aisner J, Whitacre M, Van Echo DA, et al: Combination chemotherapy for small cell carcinoma of the lung: Continuous versus alternating non-cross resistant combinations. Cancer Treat Rep 1982; 66:221.

27. Aisner J: Alternating chemotherapy for the treatment of small cell carcinoma of the lung. In: Proc 13th International Congress on Chemotherapy. SY70/4, 1983; 205:16

28. Vindelov LL, Hansen HH, Gersel A, et al.: Treatment of small cell carcinoma of the lung monitored by sequential flow-cytometric DNA-analysis. Cancer Res 1981; 42:2499.

29. Bunn PA, Schlam M, Gazdar A: Comparison of cytology and DNA content analysis by flow cytometery in specimens from lung cancer patients. Proc Am Assoc Cancer Res/ASCO 1980; 21:40.

30. Osterlind K, Hansen HH, Dombernowsky P, et al.: Combination chemotherapy of small cell lung cancer (SCLC) based on in vivo cell cycle analysis. Results of a randomized trial of 254 pts. Proc Am Assoc Cancer Res 1982; 23:154.

31. Aisner J, Forastiere A, Aroney R: Patterns of recurrence for cancer of the lung and esophagus. Cancer Treat Symp 1983; 2:87

32. Cox JD, Yesner RA: Causes of treatment failure and death in carcinoma of the lung. Yale J Biol Med 1981; 54:201

33. Fox RM, Woods RL, Brodie GN, et al.: A randomized study: Small cell anaplastic lung cancer treated by combination chemotherapy and adjuvant radiotherapy. Int J Radiat Oncol Biol Phys 1980; 6:1087.

34. Bunn P, Cohen M, Lichter A, et al.: Randomized trial of chemotherapy versus chemotherapy plus radiotherapy in limited stage small cell lung cancer. Proc Am Soc Clin Oncol 1983; 2:200.

35. Perez CA, Einhorn L, Oldham RK, et al.: Reporting for the Southeastern Cancer Study Group. Preliminary report on a randomized trial of radiotherapy (RT) to the thorax in limited small cell carcinoma of the lung treated with multiagent chemotherapy. Proc Am Soc Clin Oncol 1983; 2:190

36. Perry MC, Eaton WL, Ware J, et al. (CALGB): Chemotherapy with or without radiaton therapy in limited small cell cancer of the lung. Am Soc Clin Oncol 1984, p. 230.

37. Johnson RE, Brereton HD, Kent CN: Small cell carcinoma of the lung: Attempt to remedy causes of past therapeutic failure. Lancet 1976; 2:289

38. Hirsch FR, Paulson OB, Hansen HH, Vraa-Jensen J: Intracranial metastases in small cell carcinoma of the lung: correlation of clinical and autopsy findings. Cancer 1982; 50:2433

39. Cox JD, Komaki R, Byhardt RW, Kun LE: Results of whole-brain irradiation for metastases from small cell carcinoma of the lung. Cancer Treat Rep 1980; 64:957

40. Burgess RF, Burgess VF, Dibella NJ: Brain metastases in small cell carcinoma of the lung. JAMA 1979; 242:2084

41. Komaki R, Cox JD, Whitson W: Risk of brain metastasis from small cell carcinoma of the lung related to length of survival and prophylactic irradiation. Cancer Treat Rep 1981; 65:811

42. Nugent JL, Bunn PA jr, Matthews MJ, et al.: CNS metastases in small cell bronchogenic carcinoma: Increasing frequency and changing pattern with lengthening survival. Cancer 1979; 44:1885

182

43. Bunn PA, Ihde DC: Small cell bronchogenic carcinoma: A
     review of therapeutic results. In: Lung Cancer I, Livingston
     RB (ed). The Hague, Martinus Nijhoff, 1981; pp. 169

44. Bleehen NM, Bunn PA, Cox JD, et al.: Role of radiation
     therapy in small cell anaplastic carcinoma of the lung.
     Cancer Treat Rep 1983; 67:11

45. Hansen HH, Dombernowsky P, Hirsch F, et al: Prophylactic
     irradiation in bronchogenic small cell anaplastic
     carcinoma. A comparative trial of localized versus
     extensive radiotherapy including prophylactic brain
     irradiation in patients receiving combination
     chemotherapy. Cancer 1980; 46:279.

46. Aroney RS, Aisner J, Wesley MN, et al.: The value of
     prophylactic cranial irradiation given at complete remission
     in small cell lung cancer. Cancer Treat Rep 1983; 67:675

47. Rosen ST, Makuch RW, Lichter AS, et al.: Role of
     prophylactic cranial irradiation in prevention of central
     nervous system metastases in small cell lung cancer:
     Potential benefit restricted to patients in complete
     response. Am J Med 1983; 74:615

48. Livingston RB, Trauth CJ, Greenstreet RL: Small cell
     carcinoma: clinical manifestations and behavior with
     treatment. In: Small Cell Lung Cancer, Greco FA, Oldham RK,
     Bunn PA (eds), New York, Grune and Stratton, 1981; pp. 285

49. Poplin EA, Aisner J, Van Echo DA, et al.: CCNU,
     vincristine, methotrexate and procarbazine treatment of
     relapsed small cell lung carcinoma. Cancer Treat Rep 1982;
     66:1557

50. Cohen MH, Broder LE, Fossieck BE, et al.: Combination
     chemotherapy with vincristine, adriamycin, procarbazine in
     previously treated patients with small cell carcinoma.
     Cancer Treat Rep 1977; 61:485

51. Tinsley R, Comis R, DiFino S, et al.: Potential clinical
     synergy observed in the treatment of small cell lung cancer
     with cisplatin and VP16-213. Proc Am Soc Clin Oncol 1983; p.
     198

52. Evans WK, Osoba D, Feld R, et al.: VP16 and cisplatin for small cell lung cancer after failure of induction chemotherapy. Proc Am Soc Clin Oncol 1984; p. 222.

53. Batist G, Ihde DC, Zabell A, et al.: Small cell carcinoma of the lung: Reinduction therapy after late relapse. Ann Int Med 1983; 98:472

54. Matthews MJ, Rozencweig M, Staquet M, et al.: Long term survivors with small cell carcinoma of the lung. Eur J Cancer 1980; 16:257.

55. Bradley EC, Schechter GP, Matthews MJ, et al.: Erythro-leukemia and other hematologic complications of intensive therapy in long-term survivors of small cell lung cancer. Cancer 1982; 49:221

56. Radice PA, Matthews MJ, Ihde DC, et al.: The clinical behavior of "mixed" small cell/large cell bronchogenic carcinoma compared to "pure" small cell subtypes. Cancer 1982; 50:2894

57. Matthews MJ: Effects of therapy on the morphology and behavior of small cell carcinoma of the lung: a clinicopathologic study. In: Lung Cancer: Progress in Therapeutic Research, Muggia F, Rozencweig M (eds), New York, Raven Press, 1979, pp. 155

58. Johnson BE, Ihde DC, Lichter RS, et al.: Five to 10 year followup of small cell lung cancer patients disease free at 30 months: chronic toxicities and late relapse. Proc Am Soc Clin Oncol 1984, p. 218.

59. Zacharski LR, Henderson WG, Rickles FR, et al.: Effect of warfarin on survival in small cell carcinoma of the lung. JAMA 1981; 245:831

60. Chahinian AP, Ware JH, Zimmer B, et al.: Evaluation of anticoagulation with Warfarin and of alternating chemotherapy in extensive small cell cancer of the lung (CALGB). Am Soc Clin Oncol 1984, p. 225.

61. Yesner R: Classification of lung cancer histology. NEJM 1985; 312:652

62. Carney DN, Gazdar AF, Nau M, et al.: Two distinct classes of tumor cells cultured from patients with small cell lung cancer. Am Soc Clin Oncol, 1985, p. 218.

63. Little CD, Nau MM, Carney DN, et al.: Amplification and expression of the c-myc oncogene in human lung cancer cell lines. Nature 1983; 306:194.

64. Carney DN, Mitchell JB, Kinsella TV: In vitro radiation and chemotherapy sensitivity of established cell lines of human small cell lung cancer and large cell morphological variants. Cancer Research 1983; 43:2806

65. Minna JD: Recent advances of potential clinical importance in the biology of lung cancer. Proc Am Assoc for Cancer Res 1984; 15:393

66. Simms E, Gazdar AF, Abrams P, Minna JD: Growth of human small cell (oat cell) carcinoma of the lung in serum-free growth factor supplemented medium. Cancer Res 1980; 40:4356

67. Whang-Peng J, Bunn PA, Kao-Shan CS, et al.: A non-random chromosomal abnormality, del. 3p(14-23) in human small cell lung cancer (SCLC). Cancer Gen Cytogen 1982; 6:119.

68. Gazdar AP, Carney DN, Russel EK, et al.: Establishment of continuous clonable cultures of small-cell carcinoma of the lung which have amine precursor uptake and decarboxylation cell properties. Cancer Res 1980; 40:3502

69. Baylin SB, Gazdar AF, Minna JD, Shaper JH: Cell surface protein phenotype of human lung cancer in culture. Identification of common and distinguishing cell surface proteins on the membrane of different human lung cancer cell types. Proc Natl Acad Sci USA 1982; 79:4650.

70. Bunn PA, Linnoila I, Minna JD, et al.: Small cell lung cancer, endocrine cells of the fetal bronchus, and other neuroendocrine cells express the leu-7 antigenic determinant present on natural killer cells. Blood 1985; 65:764

71. Curt GA, Carney DN, Cowan KH, et al.: Unstable methotrexate resistance in human small cell carcinoma associated with double minute chromosomes. NEJM 1983; 308:199

72. Carney DN, Gazdar AF, Minna JD: In vitro chemosensitivity of clinical specimens and established cell lines of small cell lung cancer. Am Soc Clin Oncol, 1982, p. 10.

73. Carney DN, Ihde DC, Cohen MH, et al.: Serum neuron-specific enolase: a marker for disease extent and response to therapy for small cell lung cancer. Lancet, 1982; March 13:583

74. Cuttitta F, Carney DN, Mulshine J, et al.: Bombesin-like peptides can function as autocrine growth factors in human small cell lung cancer. Nature (in press).

75. Doyle LA, Martin WJ, Gazdar AF, et al.: Markedly decreased expression of class I histocompatibility antigens, protein and mRNA in human small cell lung cancer. J Exp Med (in press).

76. Funa K, Gazdar AF, Doyle A, et al.: In vivo induction of B_2-microglobulin on small cell lung cancer patients and mid-gut carcinoid patients treated with interferon. IV World Conference on Lung Cancer (in press).

77. Jones DH, Bleehen NM, Slater AJ, et al.: Human lymphoblastoid interferon in the treatment of small cell lung cancer. Br J Cancer 1983; 47:361

78. Mattson K, Holsti LR, Niirnen A, et al.: Human leukocyte interferon as part of a combined treatment for previously untreated small cell lung cancer. J Biol Resp Mod 1985; 4:8

SUBJECT INDEX